MW01515510

TREASURES OF DARKNESS

Hidden Riches in Secret Places

Rev. Terry [Campbell] Lebendig

xulon
PRESS

TABLE OF CONTENTS

Dedication:

This book is dedicated to Sara and all those wounded warriors, who beyond their own capabilities could not stop the abuse that became forever embedded in the memory of their souls. Their courage to tell their legend, to step into the unknown, to seek release from a lifetime of imprisonment to their wounds is unsurpassed by none.

And to my daughters who have suffered their own wounds and unconditionally loved me through the periods of darkness in my life adding to the treasures found there. Kelly, my eldest daughter, who with her strong will and determination encouraged me to write. Her sister Kristin, who as the middle child resigned herself to never receiving the recognition and attention she so richly deserved yet becoming the mom to her children, I always hoped to be. And last but never least Kari. Through her own traumatic events her faith, strength and love has grown to a level more than I could have ever hoped for.

May you never stop searching for those treasures and riches for you are all more valued than words could express and more beautiful and unique in all your ways than one could possibly imagine.   8/09/07

Preface

Recently while addressing some details with a friend in regard to an upcoming seminar, I started to reflect upon a past workshop presented by the Michigan Coalition Against Domestic and Sexual Violence held in Bellaire several years ago. In my years as a crisis counselor I have had many opportunities to attend educational seminars to increase my professional knowledge. It had not occurred to me that not only could this education enhance my professional knowledge but also bring about personal emotional healing and inspire new direction as well.

I was extremely anxious even-though I was looking forward to driving through the charming beauty of Northern Michigan headed for Shanty Creek Lodge. I literally could feel the anxiety begin to melt away as the picturesque winding roads and mammoth trees begin to enclose around me, somewhat like the arms of a mother comforting her child. The hustle and bustle of the city forgotten as the serenity of the lake water and balmy blue skies begun to settle upon me. I drove through the well known scenic main street of the village of Bellaire. It is the seat of Antrim County with a population of just greater than 1000 people at that time. Certainly a contrast, to my hometown for sometimes I felt as though that many people alone lived in my home community. Each time I travel up north, I understand the adjective "Water Wonderland" more distinctly as I bask in the tranquility of the lakes surrounding me. The deeper I traveled into the wooded area the more tranquil and picturesque the scene. I had a million dollar view of Lake Bellaire and miles of pristine hardwood forests. And I thought this was going to be a lackluster week.

Immediately, I sought out my room and was applauding myself for choosing to pay the single-rate so I did not have to share this paradise with anyone, at least not for now. I thought I had died and gone to heaven. However, I was there for a purpose not a vacation and in a few hours registration would commence to initiate five days of education. Though I did not know it at the time a week of self-realization as well. From the first session it was obvious that self-exploration and identification would be a process that would continue throughout the coming days.

From our first speaker my awareness of the vast world of tragic relationships plagued by violence broadened through her personal testimony and video clips. Until that point in my life, my view was limited to my own experiences and I knew I had begun an adventure of a lifetime. Throughout the next five days I listened to individuals tell their compelling stories of physical and emotional abuse that eventually led them or those they knew to tragic coping mechanisms such as: Drug addiction, occultism and suicide.

The poignant dramas that were unfolding made such a personal impact that it was a turning point in my life. Up to this time, I worked with alcoholics and drug addicts empathizing with the tragic environments that led them to their choices in life. I had personally experienced controlling and sometimes violent situations as a child and young married adult but had not known of the overwhelming fear and humiliation of sexual violation that brings a person to the brink of suicide. Nor my own deep imprisoned need to release my burning desire to tell those who are hurting there is a way out of their heart-ache and pain! I found it that week.

I found my own areas of vulnerability and rage. I found a determination that though deterred and distracted for far too many years cannot now be stifled! I found though scarred by past experiences God can lead you to treasures of darkness and show you riches hidden in secret places. In that unforgettable picturesque setting I found a blazing fire within my heart that won't be quenched, a journey just begun.

In the following pages I will take you on a journey through my life and the lives of victims of physical and sexual violence, addiction, abuse and eventually healing. These are true violations, true victims and true victories. Come take the journey with me the treasure of darkness you find, just may be your own.

Introduction

As a past substance abuse and sexual assault counselor, I have had the advantage and opportunity to listen to the inspiring heartfelt stories of many women and men who have been victims of abuses of diverse varieties. In addition, promoting seminars that have developed for some into transformational experiences as they as victims altered their lives by breaking the silence.

I personally have experienced some of the same difficulties and stumbling blocks along my own life's journey. I know what it is to be beaten, broken, rejected or abandoned. One of those chosen to be wounded to heal. I have sat on both sides of a therapy room. As a victim and as a counselor as many wounded warriors struggled to unlock the secrets of their past. Nothing is more rewarding than watching the light of revelation revealed on a victim's face as they recognize the fact that they are not alone in their suffering. The realization that others have suffered some of the same periods of darkness and hopelessness.

Occasionally, at a seminar there is an instantaneous transformation; more often than not it takes months of counseling. The "revelation light" experiences are no minute things, sudden but not momentary. Fortunately, they are long-lasting. My experiences, God's revelations, and the open vulnerable willingness of others to "break the silence" has brought this life-long dream to a reality.

I have invited others to share the secrets of their pasts. This is my story this is their story, a story of fear and courage, a story of tragedy and triumph and a story of wounded shattered-hearts healed by the Balm of Gilead. Some of them have written their story in their own words. They are definitely heartfelt truths that I know will touch your heart and maybe change your life. Some of the stories come from my own pain, and others directly or indirectly with permission from individuals who have shared at my seminars or in my office. We all have chosen to break the silence in order to heal within and with the hope that the sharing of experiences will assist in helping others to the same freedom.

In the following pages as you experience our suffering, our hope and finally our victory, you may or may not recognize yourself. I am willing to bet however, that there will be several stories that will reveal and crystallize your own hidden truths. So begin your journey. Laugh, cry, grow with us and discover the treasures of darkness.

Part One

Treasures of Darkness

Chapter One

Deep Waters

Isaiah 45:3 " I will give you the treasures of darkness; riches stored in secret places, so that you may know that I am the Lord, the God of Israel, who summons you by name"

Imagine feeling as though you were spiraling downward, sinking into the depths of darkness never to surface again. No one to pull you to safety, rescue or hear your cries. You feel completely alone as if drowning in despair. You feel frantic and hopeless. Though feelings cannot always be relied upon, there are times when they seem incredibly real. I have experienced that lost, lonely hopelessness in times of past heartbreak and misfortune. A desperation so profound I thought I would never ascend from the deep again. How *do* you ascend from the deep waters? How do you turn tragedies into triumphs or make your way back from devastating loss? How do you find the treasure of darkness?

My first real-life deep water experience was a literal near drowning at approximately age five. After sinking toward the bottom the third time and desperately looking for something concrete to grab onto, I began to claw and thrash my way to the surface. Do you know the more you struggle the worse it is? I know, as a child jumping into the Chandler Park Adult Pool by mistake. The more I panicked the worse it became and my thrashing to no avail. What saved my life? I became too exhausted to fight a moment longer and just let go. To this day, I remember it vividly as I let go I floated to the top and even at that young age I knew someone had been watching over me. I climbed out confused, embarrassed, shaking and wet running to the dressing room to change. No one knew of my mistake or my near death experience but to this day I am still afraid of deep water!

Throughout our lifetime we often find ourselves in deep waters, maybe leaping there out of ignorance or stubbornness. Maybe we have been pushed or never know how we ended up there. Time and time again I have learned that in the deep the best way to surface is to let go. Let go relax and just surface. In other words I learned to let go and let God, allowing his loving hands to reach in and pull me to the surface. Sometimes as you let go things will automatically change and other times it takes a miracle, the divine supernatural extraordinary intervention of God.

Have you ever needed a miracle?

Have you ever just known in your heart of hearts that the only way out of the mess you were in was beyond your power? Or stumbling into the deepest darkest area of your soul that even with all the knowledge that you could possibly gather together you could discover no answer. You needed an outside intervention. Perhaps a miracle, I have. Have you known the way of drowning maybe not literally but drowning in shame or despair. Have you suffered the pang of abandonment or the disgust of an incestuous relationship, the fear of violence. The victims of the following stories have, but we have also recognized treasures that were once hidden.

My journey through darkness began as a very young child. Though I knew it not at the time, it appears the hand of God was upon me all my life. He stepped in for the father who had abandoned me and the mother who was too broken to nurture me. His next intervention in my life occurred around the age of seven. My grandparents were raising me and that in itself must have been a divine intervention. They had removed me from my mother's care, after finding me home alone. Perhaps a treasure I was too young to distinguish in the darkness of my life. Apparently, my mother had decided it was time for her to begin to act like a mom and wanted to, intervention took place and I was legally allowed to live with my grandparents.

The treasure that I can now perceive from that terrifying moment of my childhood? The intervention by God to place me with Faith-Believing grandparents who reared me in a Christian home. Who taught me about a loving God at a time when I thought there must be something wrong with a child whose own parents would abandon her. Yes, I began my life experiences in deep waters in the shadows of darkness but it took many years for me to find the treasure and the hidden riches. Never-the-less I see now it was the intervention of God and none the less a miracle.

It took a few years to become secure in my safety, many days I watched over my shoulder after overhearing conversations that my mother was threatening to come and get me. I would run the five blocks home from school every afternoon in terror watching the streets for her red car. Then the day came, terror rose in my heart as I froze in my tracks. There it was the huge Pontiac sitting on the wrong side of the street where there was no parking. You couldn't miss it. I see it like it was just yesterday, I started to shake and stopped dead in my tracks I couldn't decide what to do. Turn around and run or head home. My cousin was with me and somehow we decided to move forward and entered the house. Hearing loud angry voices as we did so.

My mother who had been physically abused at times was no stranger to aggression herself. As we came in the door the one thing I remember to this day is my grandfather pushing us toward the kitchen. Blocking her from grabbing me, he whispered, "Go out the back door, over the fence and meet me on the next street, hide in the bushes till I get there." We did what we were told, I do remember hopping the fence, I do remember being terrified as I peeked through the bushes watching for his old Chevrolet to ramble up the street and fearing it would be the red Pontiac. I remember ending up at my Aunt Ruth's house in Dearborn and her trying to comfort me with a little red with white polka dot clown doll. I remember going back to court and finally staying with my grandparents.

I was fortunate but some of you reading this may not have been. You may have been reared by that alcoholic father or step-father and not only reared by him but abused, verbally criticized at every move you made. Laughed at, made fun of, put down, shoved around or beaten. Maybe your dad left at a young age like mine, but no one came to rescue you, leaving you with a grief-stricken or dysfunctional mother. Maybe you felt like Cinderella, put upon, left behind with more responsibility than a child should have to carry and criticized when expectations were not met. Or worse yet maybe you were violated in the most humiliating manner ever. Womanhood stripped from you before it even blossomed by a self-serving child molester. If that is the case the wounds sink deep into your heart buried and possibly yet untapped.

Read on wounded one, the stories that follow may give you insight and hope. You may identify with the humiliation or the pain, the shame or the guilt, the rage or the denial but my prayer is you will emerge from that cocoon of darkness a beautiful butterfly with a whole new world to explore. We will not drag you from that cocoon before you are ready. Our hope is that as you read story after story you will identify, you will grow and you will become ready to leave the cocoon and merge to freedom as you have never known. Become the beautiful butterfly and soar and explore as you were meant to do. Searching each beautiful flower and embracing each new aroma available. Speaking of the butterfly. I cannot help but think of Sara when I think of a cocoon of darkness and the beautiful emergence of the butterfly. That image describes her story so exquisitely.

Chapter Two

Prelude to Sara's Story

I can still recall the first day she walked into my office, an aroma of fresh perfume buoyantly filling the air around her. Her well-groomed golden blond hair lay softly at the nape of her neck and flipped back from her face almost in defiance. She walked with a set determination as if to sustain control. A behavior she fought incredibly hard to maintain through the years I counseled with her. I remember initially thinking she couldn't possibly be a victim she was too well held together. I later discovered most of the abused women I counseled hid behind that well structured pretense. Of course that is the explanation, a simulation of pretense.

Victims of abuse often take the so-called road less traveled, becoming over achievers. Displaying control on the outside while dying little-by-little daily on the inside. She sat in the comfortable chair across from me glancing around the room as if looking for some means of escape. Finding none, she locked eyes with mine as I made every attempt to portray with them the concern and care I felt for her at that moment. My job was to create an atmosphere of trust and security to someone who had not felt those emotions for years.

I went through the usual crisis-counseling routine with explanation of the program, the resources that we had to offer, a boring list of my credentials and what my role was. Then with as much gentleness as I was capable of; I turned the hour over to her with assurance that she need only to share as much information as she was comfortable with. In an non-emotional matter-of-fact manner Sara began her story, one that I will never forget!

She had been a victim she told me initially, I later discovered not once in her life but several times. She had come from a strict religious background of a particular denomination which I choose not to disclose. Quite chaotic, she had made many attempts to overcome her past and begin a new life. Attempting to bury the old one and bind it in chains for a time, that resolve broke suddenly for her one Summer day on her way to run last minute errands. As I recall, *I* began to feel victimized as her voice shook with overwhelming emotion during her detailed account of what had occurred.

Sara had come in to the crisis center to seek help following a recent brutal rape by a stranger. Though stranger rape comprises only 1-2% of the 1.3 rapes occurring every hour against women in America. Sara was one of them. Suddenly this well-groomed somewhat controlled individual became before my very eyes a wounded child. Spiritually and emotionally broken and bleeding inside, my heart began to ache for her as I struggled within me to maintain my professionalism. I desperately wanted to run to her side gather her in my arms and rock away her pain. I discovered that day and in the days to follow with many victims that all the training goes right out the window when you sit with these women and listen to the humiliating violations they suffered. You cannot help but become bonded with them. *I* believe it is even necessary in order to walk them through to victory.

She told me of a somewhat warm Summer day, when a sick depraved man reeking of alcohol stole her dignity, her honor and for a time her resolve. Beaten physically, brutalized emotionally and violated sexually she was left perhaps to die in her vehicle. But we believe a divine power, we know as God had a plan and a better purpose for her life. Somehow Sara found the courage that day to get up drive home and begin a long journey, step by agonizing step through reality to take back her life!

You may ask why did she go home, why didn't she call the police, or at least the security guard of the department store? Why didn't she go to the hospital, or at least her doctor? Why? The reason most rape victims don't. Shame, guilt, fear, shock. Most of the rape crimes in

America today are not reported for these very reasons and as a result most of the perpetrators go unpunished. Rape is called "the most underreported violent crime in America." In a large national survey of American women, only 16% of the rapes (approximately one out of every six) had ever been reported to the police according to *Rape in America: A Report to the Nation, National Victim Center, 1992.*

Through the many months that followed I sat with her in that room, I witnessed her laugh, cry, tremble with emotion and desperately fight down her rage. I sometimes prayed with her through the anger, humiliation, hope, and fear. I wish at this point that I could tell you that Sara came out on top, but the years of pain take their toll on the physical body as well as the mind and emotions. Courageous, she struggled incessantly trying to sort reality from fantasy so often a difficult task for victims of abuse. Physically there have been illnesses directly related to the rape and some more than likely to the years of stress. Today, many years later I still have contact with Sara as we work together on Seminars for Wounded Hearts. I have her permission to tell her story. I also have her permission to include her self-written recollections of the events of her violations. But beware in the next chapter her journey through violation and fear is graphic and heart-breaking.

I know she still struggles to defeat the battle the enemy so precariously has placed in her path by testifying to the victories she has attained. She faces the reality today that in the past she struggled so desperately to escape. Escape from reality is often a common defense mechanism used by victims of incest and rape.

I recall her describing in great detail a picture on the wall of her bedroom. A small cottage located in a meadow with a path of flowers leading to a wooden doorway. She explained that she would stare at the picture. She would imagine herself on the path stopping to smell the sweet aroma of flowers leading to the doorway becoming immersed in the safety of the serene little cottage while her body was violated by her attacker. I remember that at the time it was all I could do to hold back my tears and maintain some semblance of professionalism. There were moments when unsuccessful, I would let the tears flow slowly silently down my cheeks and fight desperately to keep my emotion hidden from her.

A child of incest lies in fear and trepidation, night after night apprehensively awaiting the footsteps of her violator. Their heart races, their palms sweat as nausea rises within them. When the fear becomes reality, the mind transfers the reality to fantasy. A child may learn to retreat to a place where many of them are unable to tell the difference. Victims learn to survive in the worst of circumstances by disassociating with reality, removing themselves from the actual circumstance for a time. The ultimate form of denial yet a way of survival. Healing from past wounds becomes difficult when the reality is reconciled with because along with reality comes the flood of anguish and the pain they originally sought to escape. The challenge for the counselor is guiding a victim in crisis by encouraging them to face the fear and then let go. Sara struggled in those first sessions to maintain her control and tested me incessantly to see just how much intimacy she could share without a judgmental reaction. I wondered if the memories were truly deeply buried or deliberately hidden until she trusted me enough to divulge. Sara certainly has had struggles that have knocked her down, bless God she always gets up and keeps pushing on. There will always be those uphill battles as Miley Cyrus sings in "The Climb", another mountain to climb. She has her battles but keeps looking for the treasures and finds them!

Chapter Three

Sara's Story

The following chapter is transcribed exactly from the written manuscript given to me personally by Sara, the events listed here are the vivid and graphic memories she recalls from her past violations as written by her.

Journey Through Fear by Sara Ylen

"A life lived in fear is a life half-lived." As those words were spoken to me for the first at the age of 30, I felt a mixture of inspiration and sorrow. Memories were flooding to the surface and all of them were associated with fear. I choked and fought back tears as I tried to wrestle these recollections into submission but to no avail. The past was going to haunt me forever at this rate. I knew it deep in my soul that day as I struggled to deny my roots. It was time to surrender and go back to the beginning once again...

Flat terrain and infinite fields of corn, navy beans and sugar beets were the characteristics of my hometown surroundings. Growing up in a small farming community had lent itself to living undetected under the domination of a controlling violent man I called "Daddy". My mother, a heart patient since birth, had chosen self-preservation over the protection of her children. Her fear gave birth to mine.

"Just wait until you father gets home." I would tremble at those words echoed in my direction, knowing that the peace of death would be preferable to what would happen when my father walked in the door. My earliest memories start at age three and no memory goes untouched by the rage of a man who wanted perfect little soldiers in his repertoire of life accomplishments. Everything seemed to anger him. As a three year-old I started sleep-walking. Each night I'd wander to an interesting place for the rest of the night's sleep. Until one night, I parked across the door-way of my parents' bedroom. My father, an early riser, tripped over me on his way down the darkened hallway. I can still her the sickening thud and feel the blinding pain as he kicked me down the hallway to the entrance of my own bedroom and left me there. Times like these were far too frequent to recount and each event escalated more than the previous one.

At the age of six, I became caretaker, mother and substitute wife. Each role fed the voracious fear that raged inside of me. By day, I was cook and cleaning lady. By night, I was captive to the diseased mind of a child molester who would, years later, be profiled as a sexual sadist. I would pray to disappear into the sunset that cast a glow on my bedroom wall while I tried to escape from the sweaty stench of my father breathing in my face and destroying my innocence. What started off as violent rape soon turned into sadistic torture. He had no conscience.

A result of his upbringing, my brother started to follow in our father's footsteps. being three years my elder, he was my best friend. Dad had isolated us from everyone and my brother was my only companion much of the time. We starved together when mom would sleep all day and demand that we stay in our rooms without food. We would hide outside in the barn together when dad was angry and searching for an outlet. We would find safe havens under bridges and catch crayfish while we pretended to be someone else's children. I respected him more than anyone. We had both been robbed of childhood as we struggled to survive in the traumatic adult world we'd been hurled into. However, the summer he turned twelve and I was nine, darkness overtook him. That summer, he became his father's son forcing me into oral sex and organizing times his friends could come over and do what they wanted to his sister. My safety net was gone. I felt abandoned by everyone.

By the time I was fifteen, I had been pregnant twice because of incest. My father would know and he would beat me within inches of death forcing miscarriage every time. All I wanted was a way out. I had tried telling friends and teachers. Social workers and police officers had questioned my father and me, documenting bruises and pregnancies. Ultimately, the monster won. Time after time, he'd convince everyone I was lying and the saving I hoped for never occurred. My childhood was half-lived. I depended on fear to survive. Those years were the roots of my sorrow.

At the tender age of eighteen, I married my first love and vowed never to look back. I would rise above my fear, perfect being a wife to a man who deserved my love and pray for the chance to raise my own children in a home that would be full of unconditional love and acceptance. Fear would not enter into our home or the hearts of my children. For eight blissful years, I enjoyed such a home. I grew as an individual, fought to leave my childhood in the past, and brought two beautiful sons into the world. Motherhood was everything I'd dreamed it to be and I dedicated my existence to giving my sons health, happiness and security. I had defeated the cycle of panic and violence and I basked proudly in the peaceful aura that encircled my children. But fear did not stay banished. It made an undesirable return to my life on May 12,2001 in the form of a stranger in a parking lot. And this time, my terror would take on a life of its own. I worried I would never be the same. The beauty of it is—I never was.

Saturday, May 12,2001 was a cliché day—sunny, not a cloud in the sky and blissfully balmy. By mid-morning, I had been transformed into a beautiful swan by a talented stylist as I described to her the dress I would be wearing for my friend's wedding the next day. My friend had entrusted me with rehearsal dinner details and a polished wedding procession. The dinner was to be that night and I was energized about it as I was in the wedding that would follow the next day. For all intents and purposes, life was perfect. All I needed were a few items from the grocery store and my plans would be complete. So I drove to the busiest, most economical store in the area. There in that parking lot as I parked my car, opened my door and reached back to grab my purse the clock struck twelve and my beautiful life disappeared.

He was there. I turned and at the same moment, I felt his hand crushing my arm. His smell: alcohol, the cigarettes and the foul "all night at the bar" odor pierced by brain quickly. He was wasting no time as he continued to crush my arm, pushing against me, swearing at me and finally laughing as I begged him to take my possessions and let me go. Instead he invaded every personal space I possessed as he pummeled my unsuspecting body, laughed as I begged for my life, raped me and left me exposed and unconscious. When consciousness finally returned, I started my long descent into the most dismal era of my life. In that instant, panic and terror had me in a steel grip, compelling me to believe that I would never be able to go on.

In my craving for safety, I drove the twenty-five miles from that parking lot to the home I shared with my husband and little boys. To this day, I have no memory of that drive home. What is etched in my memory, though, is the look on my husband's face when I stepped inside our home and let my full weight fall against our insulated door. I knew from that moment that I could never tell him the whole truth. It would kill him—break his heart—and our children couldn't afford to lose another parent. I felt as if my ability to mother was already shattered. After all, I'd promised my children on the day of their births that I would provide total and absolute protection. How could I protect them, though, when I was living in sheer terror myself?

My inability to face the truth induced denial of gargantuan proportions that allowed me to carry on a beleaguered existence. Though I tried to maintain normalcy, the truth was never far under the surface and little by little, I knew I had to start facing it. I had shared enough of my truth with my husband to explain my physical injuries. So when, forty-eight hours after my attack, I decided to contact the police, I only shared those same details with the investigating officer. Incident report number in hand, I repeated this performance for the emergency room physician assigned to care for the muscle and nerve damage to my neck, left arm, shoulder and displaced ribs and pelvic bones.

"Sara, you have to tell your husband." It was the Tuesday after my assault and I had broken my silence over a steak and baked potato. The steak turned to rubber and my throat closed as my trusted confidante stared into my startled eyes. I had just described to her in sketchy terms the moment before I faded into unconsciousness for the second time, when "the man" had slid his gold nugget and diamond ring onto the knuckle of his middle finger. Through clenched teeth he swore at me and vowed to shut me up as he forced that ring and finger inside my body. She hadn't even heard the most horrible component of my defilement—the second rape. But already she was making demands. My body was throbbing with pain, my abdomen cramped and I could smell his scent as nausea washed over me in vicious waves.

"I can't," was my edgy response. However, her facial expression spoke volumes and I knew that before the day was over I would comply. That night, as I struggled to find the words, I reached the same threshold with my husband that I had earlier that day at lunch. I couldn't go beyond that first violation. His reaction to just that portion of my reality was more than either of us could handle. Adrenalin took over as I ran from room to room, locking windows and doors, closing curtains and making repeated checks that all points of entry were locked and protected. My fear had just escalated into hysteria.

"Do you think I want this to be true? I don't It would be so much easier.." Pain enveloped my body and cut off my air mid-sentence. I fell to the floor sobbing. Night-time settled in and agony became my companion as searing pelvic pain and abnormal bleeding overtook me. By morning, I was begging my husband to return me to the emergency room. I wanted him to believe. I wanted someone to tell me I was going to be okay. I wanted to surrender to the capable hands of a doctor and nurse who understood that rape was a living hell.

No such professional existed, however. Despite my inner pleading, there was no peace or resolution. The doctor and nurse took turns reprimanding me for the egregious mistake of waiting too long to come forward.

"Rape kits are useless past seventy-two hours, Mrs. Ylen." The word "useless" flashed through my mind like a neon sign. Synonyms inundated my brain—expendable, hopeless, worthless, weak, inadequate and futile. Yes, those words seemed inadequate. It was time to admit that's what I was. I decided then and there that I would be forever broken.

For several agonizing months, I struggled just to move past the physical wounds I'd been left with. Pain killers and muscle relaxers became my favored companions. I watched my children build their own walls of fear. At night, my four year-old angel would pray for "the bad man" to leave his mommy alone. As my physical pain slowly started to subside, I was left with the startling reality that the deepest wounds were yet to be faced and that was an impossible task. It meant admitting pain, violation, betrayal and what those things had done to my self-worth.

"One day at a time, Sara," was everyone's catch phrase as if it carried the cure I was seeking. But one day was too much. One hour was too much. I had to live minute to minute. Nothing else seemed achievable. Each day I woke up in a cloud of despair, feeling abandoned by pretty much everyone in my life and worrying that my children were being eternally affected by my nagging self-doubt and misery. Life was desultory and meaningless. Inside me something was screaming to get out, but there was no clearly marked exit. Little did I know that it was a warrior who wanted out and the next person I met would name her "Xena".

Thirteen months after my rape, the first of several first-rate police officer came into my life. As a Sergeant for the Michigan State Police and as a survivor of child sexual abuse, she extended an invitation to me if I should ever wish to talk. Expecting that she would scold me as did everyone before her; I contemplated her offer with trepidation. With nothing to lose, I finally walked into her place of employment and started the journey that would turn things around. For two uninterrupted hours, she sat across from me as I stumbled and stammered my way through the telling. I wanted to understand but my vocabulary didn't include the phrase "I was raped." Finally, she put her hand up and I stopped speaking.

"Sara, you were raped," she said slowly and methodically, letting it pierce my subconscious. "You can't deny that anymore. He got a piece of you. But he didn't get all of you. The pieces that are left are pretty good. So fight for them!" Fight for them? She spoke with such conviction and fervor that something inside me immediately shifted.

"You can do it, Sara. I will believe in you until you believe in you." Her statements were laconic but her intent was clear. She would be my teacher, instructing me in the highly coveted art of reclaiming myself by going to war for what was rightfully mine.

Within days, my trust in her direction was put to the test. As I drove to a doctor's appointment, I passed a vehicle waiting to pull out in traffic. The driver was a man— one who strongly resembled my attacker. He entered traffic behind me and as my panic-stricken heart raced, I studied this man in my rearview mirror. He raised his left hand to run his finger through his long hair and on his middle finger was a ring. The pounding in my head kept time with my heart as my body braced for another attack and throbbed in remembrance of the first one. Numb and immobile, I sat in the parking lot of my doctor's office not knowing how I got there. "The pieces that are left are pretty good, Sara. Fight for them." I wanted to fight but I didn't know how. What I did know is that my fear was larger than life and if I did nothing then I would be looking over my shoulder for the rest of my life. I didn't deserve that. More than that, my children didn't deserve that.

My next stop was at my therapist's office where I choked out every facet of my traffic scare and expressed my longing to fight back. Within minutes, I was in my therapist's car heading toward the driveway "he" had pulled out of earlier that morning. Armed with an address, I placed a phone call to the original investigating officer. His shock that I would call him over a year later was unmistakable.

And so my journey through the criminal justice system began. It would be measured in months of peaks and valleys. Four full days would be spent looking through eight thousand mug shots of white males that led to my attacker's undeniable identification, only to fail weeks later at picking him out of a corporal lineup because he'd completely changed his appearance. Outstanding detectives would discover a pawn shop record that led back to the man I identified, verifying he'd pawned a ring matching my description just four days after raping me. Employment records would establish that he was an employee of the store where the crime occurred and that he was at work that fateful day. I provided a description of a skull tattoo on my attacker's right bicep and the man from the mug shot possessed that exact tattoo. The case was inundated with delays but ultimately, in March of 2003, James Eugene Grissom—the man who destroyed pieces of my life—was arrested and charged with two counts of first degree criminal sexual conduct, each bearing up to life in prison as a penalty.

New emotions, positive ones overwhelmed me—feelings of power, security, victory and freedom. These feelings were ephemeral though, as I tried to reconcile the desire to see it through with the dread of facing this man in court. Confronted with reliving every grisly, lurid detail in front of a judge and jury, I felt fragmented and uncertain. However, once again what I most feared was the very thing that strengthened and transformed me.

My friend, the Sergeant had been there with me through all the ups and downs. She willingly graced me with the benefits of her professional and personal experience and I could feel something decisive growing inside me. As I described each personal battle that arose while waiting for the trial, suddenly a smile spread across her face. "You've got it, Sara. You found the warrior princess inside you and I, for one, don't want to mess with Xena. So when you feel like you're going to lose, let Xena take over and you'll be fine."

After numerous pretrial motions and postponements, the felony trial finally started on August 19,2003. With the help of greatly trusted professionals, I had exerted tremendous effort in preparing myself for testifying. This had to be the moment where I spoke my truth without fearing the man who had created it. I wanted to be real—connected to the pain that I was going to describe—for only then could I truly be heard.

The trial was spread out over a period of eight days and the night before I was going to take the stand, I snuggled with my boys in front of the television. As we watched a movie together, the dialog grabbed hold of my psyche when I heard a character say: Courage is not the absence of fear, but rather the judgment that there is something more important than fear." The inner halcyon that suddenly set in raised my awareness. This was the answer—courage. I could get through testifying if I decided that telling my truth was more important than living in dread.

"Please state your full name for the court and spell your last name." I inhaled sharply as my moment of truth began with this by-the-book exchange. For two and one-half hours, I bore witness to the gruesome acts committed against me and defied the entrapment of the defense attorney. In the end, the judge and jury saw James Eugene Grissom through my eyes—as a singularly repugnant man. More importantly, as I stepped off the stand and release all of the agony I had been carrying for two years, the truth had set me free. My attacker was in jeopardy and his fear glistened in his eyes and glowed in ghastly white skin. From that point on, I knew there was going to be more fear in my life. There would be hope. I felt it with every fiber of my being.

Five days after testifying, the trial finally ended. Less than an hour of deliberation sent two "guilty" verdicts echoing through the courtroom. Stepping outside of the courthouse that day, my ebullience peaked and so my journey into healing accelerated. That night, as I celebrated my personal triumph, I hugged my boys tightly. My oldest son saw my perpetual smiles and wondered why I was different.

"You don't have to pray for that bad man to leave me alone anymore, honey. The bad man got told he's going to prison." He threw his arms around me as his own little face lit up. "For how long, Mommy? Forever?"

"I don't know. The judge will have to decide that in a few weeks."

"I hope he goes to prison for a million-billion-trillion years, Mom."

"Me too, honey. Me too."

Ultimately, the judge rewarded my survival and truth-telling by exceeding the sentencing guidelines and sending my rapist to prison for fifteen to thirty-five years. What a remarkable victory! However, the greater triumph in all of this has been the journey of reclaiming me. I had lived far longer than I wanted to admit believing that I was worthless. Malevolent shadows had surrounded so much of my life that I was convinced it was all I could lay claim to. However the alchemy of being a rape survivor is that it has the power to make you so much stronger than you can ever imagine—if you let it.

One of my first conversations with a fellow rape survivor had introduced just such a concept. She was four years past her rape and she told me if I just trusted the process, someday I would be grateful for what happened to me. I rolled my eyes and determined instantly that she was insane. How could someone ever be grateful for violation and betrayal? Now, as I approach the six year anniversary of my rape, I understand.

Life is not merely what happens to you. It is what you carry inside of you as you walk through each moment. I never would have appreciated this if not for my life experiences. For a long time I would repeat the courage mantra from the movie, all the while feeling like courage was fleeting. As I stepped into the public eye and told my persona story so that others might be helped, I heard people refer to me as "brave" and "strong". I rejected those portrayals, not believing that I deserved such honorable titles.

Today though, I can say "thank you" and know there is more than fear and uncertainty. I have the satisfaction of knowing that I have fought battles in the past two years that I never would have approached were it not for the experience that caused my personal awakening.

Triumphantly, I have fought back even against my father. He knows, now, that I will not be silent any longer. Though he remains a free man instead of a condemned criminal, I take steps every day to be free of the memories that haunt me. Each sadistic trauma he inflicted is a measurement of who he is— not who I am. The are pieces of me. They don't define me.

Even now, I battle cancer that threatens to destroy me. But, I will not live half of a life because of fear. Surrender is no longer an option. What I now carry inside me is hope, determination and peace— the hope that I will be able to keep learning, the determination to be true to what is important and the peace knowing that my children will never again lose their mother to a madman. E.E.

Cummings said it best when saying this: "To be nobody-but-your-self-in a world, which is doing its best, night and day, to make you everybody else- means to fight the hardest battle which any human being can fight; and never stop fighting."

Chapter Four

Slamming the Door on Victimization
{With Reflections from Survivors}

I n sharing with you earlier I mentioned that Butterflies and Cocoons bring pleasant thoughts to mind of Sara. The struggle so immensely necessary to bring forth their beauty and freedom. Our present sufferings cannot weigh against the glory that will be revealed through them.

I have heard told more than once stories of those who have attempted to contain a moth, one specifically was an emperor moth. The story goes that in keeping a cocoon, this particular one very unusual in its construction for it had a narrow opening through which it is designed so the mature insect may force its way to escape, an immense catastrophe occurs. One of the accounts that I have been told notes that it would seem impossible for the bulky insect to make its way through the miniature opening. Having visualized a cocoon myself I can see the great discrepancy of the task at hand. Obviously, it would take a great deal labor and difficulty to accomplish.

It is believed by scientists that the pressure against the swollen body of the moth as it passes through the narrow opening is nature's way of forcing fluid into the undeveloped wings. Those that have tried in their own way to hurry the process, or assist the imprisoned creature to escape have done so with dire consequence. The moth will yes, escape and crawl out; however with a swollen body and shriveled wings! Misplaced impatience or tenderness proves to be its demise, never to become the beautiful butterfly soaring in freedom. An aborted destiny.

I think of this butterfly with sorrow as it reminds me of all those who are struggling with suffering and sorrow. My tendency would be to rush to their deliverance immediately and assist them out of their entrapment and how do I know but that these trials of faith may contain treasures of darkness. How do I know but that perfect love seeks perfection far above their momentary suffering bringing glory through their tribulation. How do I know that were I to assist them too quickly they would emerge a swollen being unable to take flight.

Often, once becoming a victim of any type of abuse unfathomable memories form. Previously buried deep into the recesses of our mind they surface from time to time like a whale bursting forth onto the surface of the Sea. Recollections though hazy at times and unclear are still painful and may surface voluntarily or involuntarily. As the victim meditates upon these memories unexpected pain may surface with such a sudden force that it threatens their very existence. However more often than not, they are shoved with a vengeance once again into the deep recesses of our mind only to rear their hideous selves at unforeseen times or unexplainable manifestations. These memories sometimes define who we are and we let them. It is far better to not allow the past to determine who we are but rather who we become.

Letting the past victimization determine our future is a set up to repetitive victimization. Changing the course of our lives requires letting go once and for all and closing the door. Slamming the door on victimization requires courage, knowledge, and inner strength that is beyond us. Only a power greater can enable us to overcome what so often threatens to devastate us. The 12-Step Program of Alcoholics Anonymous refers in its first step to our powerlessness. Throughout those steps to overcoming addictive mindsets it refers to changing our thinking, letting go of those things of the past. The Bible in *Proverbs 23:7 KJV says: "As he thinks in his heart, so is he"*. If we continue to think we are victims then we are. Determination to remove old mindsets and replace them with new is the goal and the door handle to slamming it shut forever.

Decision and Determination first requires recognition. Reaching for the Handle is the first step but Why, What and How do I reach the handle to slam the door shut? We tend to judge and discredit ourselves by carrying the weightiness of unworthiness; embracing the mindset that somehow we are worthless. Carrying little self-respect we project the same image to the world around us, arousing the appetite of our spiritual enemy as well as those he works through in the natural world. It is as if on the assembly line we have been stamped: "Reject, spoiled goods!"

We carry the assumption that we deserve nothing better than what we have always received and nothing better will come our way. Thus the self-fulfilling prophecy pattern begins. With such a self-defeating mindset, we continue to be defeated. We attract those who want to exploit and conquer, so concluding that everyone is out to get us. Even God, *if* we recognize *He is* then we blame him. We believe He has deserted us and is therefore untrustworthy. After all, where was God when we needed protection from the traumatizing insane violation, so why would we think he would empower us to heal from the effects? In the deepest recesses of my heart I remember times of allowing just that kind of "stinkin thinkin" to set in and thus the pattern of abuse began. Can you relate? Have you had periods of stinkin thinkin, that self-defeating mindset?

In my years, of personal abuse survival and subsequent inter-action with abuse victims, I have yet to meet a "one-timer". The person who is victimized and never falls into the pattern again. Not of course, to suggest they do not exist but merely to point out that recidivism is the norm. The more we attract and respond to abuse the more abuse we receive. Statistics actually show that the person with a loving nurturing personality is attracted to a person who needs fixing. More often than not the person in need is dys-functional and controlling. The attraction is the desire to solve the dysfunction and soften the hardened personality. Involvement in this pattern is a mere distraction from the destiny God has designed for us. Everything we project says "Victim resides here, welcome please enter". The downward spiral begins leading to isolation and/or depression. Negative feeling, thus negative speaking and finally negative action follows. The more you speak it the more you believe it! Stinkin thinkin voiced begets actions setting forth patterns that develop the character. The pattern of abuse usually continues until the consequences warrant desperate measures. Then we reach for the handle, the first step in slamming the door shut on victimization!

Cheer up though, it is time for redirection, restoration, and revitalization of your life. You can be rescued from the tangled web of destruction. God can and will rescue you, you think he can't? I am here to tell you in addition to the others who have contributed to these writings. He definitely can! You think He won't? He will! In reading this book you will bear witness as individuals, as well as myself, openly share stories of overcoming, consequently slamming their own doors shut forever! You can make a decision now at this very instant or later if you so choose. The power is within you, reach for the handle of that door, take a deep breath and get ready to slam the door shut forever! Change your victim status now to victorious! **Why?** *Romans 8:37 "Nay in all these things we are more than conquerors through him that loved us."KJV* **Where?** *Ephesians 4:23"And be renewed in the spirit of your mind." and* **How?** Surrender, turn it over now, give it to God. *Proverbs 3:5 "Trust in the LORD with all thine heart; and lean not unto thine own understanding." KJV*

If this is a difficult task for you, you don't have a relationship with God or if you have blamed God, then talk with Him about it. Relationships begin with communication. If you are angry then put the blame where it really belongs on the one who prowls in the spiritual realm seeking whom he may devour. The enemy!

I know that the Lord knows your pain. You may know that, but have difficulty putting it into practice or you may not yet believe it. Either way, He suffered as much and more than you did. He was beaten unto blood, persecuted, abandoned, violated and unheard and finally crucified. Hold not ought against the power to set you free. He says in His word, He will never leave nor forsake you. He is waiting just as He was for me and for others.

There were times when I did not believe as I do today. The most bewildered I ever felt followed one of the traumatic events in my life. Where was God then? I questioned my pastor at the time and her answer to me, "What God has permitted, He has allowed." Unable to accept such an answer *at the time*, I stowed it away in the recesses of my mind until I could grasp and accept it. When I finally understood the depth of that statement I realized that yes, God had been there all the time. Grieving as I grieved, angry at the circumstance right along with me, filling me with grace I could not comprehend but sufficient to carry me through the circumstance. Much like a parent who allows difficult circumstances in a child's life that must not be interfered with; full well knowing they will be uncomfortable but later will assist in the development of their child's character.

He is waiting even now. Don't wait for him to release you from your bondage, He is waiting for you to release His power in your situation. Don't fall into the trap of repression, regression, addiction, or aggression to deal with your pain. Open the door of repentance as you walk through the following chapters of forgiveness, understanding, willingness, and healing. Learn the warfare necessary to "SLAM THE DOOR ON VICTIMIZATION".

Reflections From Survivors
From Darkness to Light
Written by: Ashleigh Lynne Chmiola

Have you ever thought it was ok to get walked on, treated like your nothing, honestly? Look at your life and imagine yourself out of your body and looking at you, no one else just you. What do you see? Well, I'm Ashleigh Chmiola and I'm going to tell you how my life has changed completely and what I used to see, what I see now, and what I am looking forward to seeing. Back when I was a young girl I had an amazing life better than I could ever imagine and then the worst thing imaginable happened, something unbelievable. Something you couldn't imagine happening to anyone, especially a young girl. Trust me, I know because I didn't expect it to happen to me and it did.

It was the summer of 2004 and I was babysitting for a friend of my mothers, Mrs. Dawn. I had watched her son occasionally throughout the summer. This particular day she had to work in the morning and run a couple of errands afterwards and that she'd be running a little late. We waited for her patiently playing games, watching movies and baking cookies but Shane, her son wanted to go swimming. I don't blame the kid it was a hot day. So I told him, "Wait until your mom gets home and then we will go swimming."

When Mrs. Dawn came home she decided to take us all swimming; me, my brother, my sister, Shane & herself. Well my mom didn't want us going alone so my step dad Pete went with us. We all walked down laughing and giggling anxious to get in the pool. We all talked about how we were going to get in jumping, cannon ball, kick flip.

We were having a great time with all of our friends swimming, jumping, playing chicken like the summer should be. Well, my little sister had to go to the bathroom so my step-dad left and took her. Mrs. Dawn happened to be scolding her son for something he had done, and then *it happened,* the moment that would change my life completely and I mean a complete one-eighty turn around.

One of the guys, my step dad had been talking to earlier, none of us really knew the guy other than his name was David. He was throwing all of us kids into in the pool and I wanted to be thrown too. so I swam over to him expecting that and instead I got a wet slimy gross hand down the bottoms of my swimsuit. I quickly swam away kicking him while doing it. I was so disgusted with my self how could I let such a disgusting and terrible thing happen to me. I had walked home quietly thinking to myself I had just been sexually assaulted. At the time I didn't know what it was other then my grandma taught a class on it.

So when I got home I went to my room and thought about it. What to do? Should I say something? How do I tell my parents? I eventually went down stairs and talked to my mom about it. At first she was like why didn't you tell me as soon as you got home but then realized how scared I was. When I told her she immediately called the cops and made me sit at the kitchen table and told me how I was going to have to tell the cops everything and it had to be the absolute truth. As the cops arrived at my house it became the center of attention.

A couple years have now gone by and I have dealt with the numerous struggles of an ordinary teenager but mine, well, they always came harder because I had God on my side. Through these difficult times we face a lot. Some of us believe there is no way out but there really is a way and it is through God. I go through my ups and downs with the struggles of Satan throwing things at me.

Sexual Assault is a difficult situation to overcome and even talk about sometimes and even for me its extremely difficult to write about. My life has completely changed since the incident. As I look at myself in the past, I see a young girl struggling with her focus and someone wanting so hard to try and break through her broken skin of the hurt and confused. Wanting so hard to become the real teenager everyone and she wants to be. How he was a pervert who had no right doing what he did to her and that she was ok and he was wrong and needs help. Now I see a teenager who wants to show the world she's different now and the power of God can move her in many ways if she's not afraid to let him move her.

I sometimes look at myself and wonder, what if I didn't go swimming? What if I decided to stay home? What if? What if? What if? Well, recently I learned from living with my Stepmom, Janet and

Dad, Tim in Virginia that you can't always live your life based on "what if" I did this, "what if" I did that? You can't always live life according to what if? Because. if you do you're not really living your life to the fullest. We have to live life as if there's no tomorrow as if you were to somehow not see the sunrise the next day.

God lets all things happen for a reason and I believe now he only let this happen to me to grow into the person I am becoming today. God loves all just the way we are, and there's nothing we can do to change that. Anything you may go through in life God is always there and he still loves you no matter what. If you get the chance open your Bible and read Ephesians Chapter 5. I read it in youth tonight and it really speaks the truth on why God is so great to you and to me.

As I looked toward my future, I was scared and didn't know what I wanted from life and all that it had out there. What am I going to do? I used to ask my self daily. Now well that's a different story, here I am less than a year from graduating and I am starting to see the amazing, smart, talented, young lady my entire family has been trying to show me and I am now really excited about my future. So you see when everything around comes down, God can always pick you back up if you let him? And now I am starting to let him pick up the broken pieces of my heart and put them together as the young woman he wants me to be.

Authors note:

Ephesians 5:8-11
"For you were once darkness, but now you are light in the Lord. Live as children of light (for the fruit of the light consists in all good-ness, righteousness and truth)and find out what pleases the Lord. Have nothing to do with the fruitless deeds of darkness, but rather expose them."

Wounded Warrior

Psalms 142:4 "Look to the right and see; for there is no one who regards me" NASB, 1995

The psalmist most poignant words quoted above could depict the inner turmoil of a little girl whose trusted authority figure has betrayed her. I witnessed as she struggled composed, now a young woman to pour out the humiliation and violation laid upon her as a child. A humiliation no human should have to endure. Splinters of shattered trust threatening her ability to relate. The enemy, her own father persecuted her soul, trampled her dreams, and crushed her spirit making her dwell in unfamiliar places. The psalmist knows he has experienced that same pain, dwelt in darkest of places.

My heart is appalled, her wounded heart wounding mine. Who could know the depths of her despair, the sting of devastation such as this? Just one: the Son who bore humiliation, rejection and separation from his own loving father.

Suddenly, one day she appears purposely driven trading ashes for beauty. There is now a raison d'être, a rationale to her suffering. She has become a paragon of virtue and integrity set forth in warfare to take back a devastated land. Empowered, if you will!

Down comes the prison's door! The key to healing has been discovered, unlocking the treasure to be found. No longer drowning in shame, drenched in fear, she is free! Sounding the alarm: "Forward March", she slaughters humiliation, lets go of the past and smashes with vengeance the inner declaration of the young wounded heart!

Victorious shouts of Praise to the one who now carries her pain within His heart and grieves for her lost innocence, inciting her to victory; drenching her now with the balm of healing. Broken, spilled out and cleansed she brings death to the waste places turning deserts into plush gardens of new growth. The enemy put to shame the wounded warrior set forth to set others free. JTC "04"

"To The Women in the world,

It is 1996, I was six years old when my dad assaulted me and his friends helped, I am 12 now. Don't let them corner you in anyway. If you have kids Please Please don't let them be around anyone you don't trust that much. Like Uncels, Brothers, dads, friends, and ect... That was how I was raped." Anonymous, 2002 {copied exactly as it was written to me.}

YESTERDAY: 1994

The sky is grey and clouded, Thunder rumbles up above. I am sad and lonely my heart rumbles too. I am left with only memories, the rains can never wash away. The beauty of a love that was ours yesterday. The leaves now have all turned color and fallen to the ground. The trees bare, the air brisk and cold; my heart shivers. Spring will come and bring the buds, sun and flowers and the memories of a love that was once was ours yesterday. Anonymous { Included with permission from a domestic violence survivor.}

LORD, I NEED A MIRACLE

I sit here writing picturing a bottle, full of dark liquid evil swirling like a cesspool. In the center, drowning, gasping for air my beloved unable to pull himself out. I am unable in any way to reach him, the force and grasp of the liquid more powerful than I. I am powerless, hours of suffering begging helpless to do anything to remove him from this hell. Alcohol the sound infuriates, nauseates me, I let go, its the only thing I can do or I will sink too. {An alcoholic's wife} "If I tell you where I'm hiding, will you promise to find me?"

CONTINUE THE RIDE

I have found my path to be long and winding with many ups and downs. Along my journey to health and healing I have been joined by many survivors. Some I have walked with a long time and some fellow travelers have been only for a season. They have blessed my life and encouraged my walk. I continue my walk of healing which I have realized will last a lifetime, but I look for those who bring peace, joy and encourage to my life. I say "continue the ride!" {wishes to remain anonymous}

LOVED TO LIVE LIFE, UNTIL—

I once was a young woman beautiful and carefree. Loved to live life, Life begun to love. Until one day I meet a man, thought one of my dreams. Until a day came, I thought God was punishing me. So in love and dared for anyone to say or think different. He became my God and I became his servant. His wish became my command and his orders I obeyed. All the while we argued, fussed and fought, not once was I happy, not even by his gentle touch. The things we once did that I used to enjoy became unexciting because of the things I endured. Being abused mentally, physically and emotionally non stop had begun to put tar on my body. I began to worry a lot and think things was my fault? Am I not pleasing? Do I say things to make him angry. My skin began to darken under my eyes, I wore bags. My hair, I did not do anymore. Laughs, was no need for them. They didn't do no good. I wore baggy clothes, jogging pants, and tee shirts. I stopped caring and loving myself, I no longer was care free. Ms. Terry has my permission to publish my writing in her book.

L. Sims

Chapter Five

Parting the Seas

I believe in miracles and I need miracles and I have experienced miracles. It was a miracle for me, just as it was a miracle when Moses parted the Red Sea and it was a miracle when "manna fell from heaven" in the wilderness. Has God ever parted a proverbial sea for you so that you could escape as the enemy pursued? Or are you in a place where you cannot yet see the interventions of God? Had God not intervened in my life as a young child, I would have been reared in that alcoholic home of abuse earlier described to you. My father an alcoholic, my mother co-dependent became an alcoholic. God defended and delivered me from the anguish of a potentially harmful situation. I was unable to see that then, all I focused on was my fear and pain. He can defend and deliver you whatever the situation. Even if it takes a miracle.

Psalm 50:15 "And call upon me in the day of trouble: I will deliver the and thou shalt glorify me" KJV

Isaiah 19:20 "It will be a sign and witness to the Lord Almighty in the land of Egypt. When they cry out to the Lord because of their oppressors, he will send them a savior and defender, and he will rescue them"

It was a miracle when Elijah met the needs of the widow of Zarephath and it was a miracle when God met the needs of a young suicidal divorcee in Cadillac after a tragic divorce that subsequently led to one of the most devastating losses of my life; custody of my children. I can honestly say that I did not yet comprehend the full meaning of hopelessness, despair and discouragement until that time in my life. My insecurities and familiarity with abandonment had left me overburdened with a heavy load of baggage. That, coupled with immaturity and inability to cope with the trials of life, a sixteen year marriage came to an end. A raging custody battle followed and I gave in, some thought I gave up I guess it is how you choose to look at it.

I came to a deep place of despair and their was no turning back. The enemy was battering me and advancing quickly, I was running for my life with a vastness spread before me much like the Red Sea was an obstacle for the Israelites. Close at my heels the whole time breathing hot upon my neck. My feeble attempts to put my life together were a disaster and led me to a dark place of despair. I was angry and yes, even angry at God. How in the world could He possibly let this happen to me, of all people? After all, I was a church-going dedicated wife and mother. The Bible warns us rain falls on the just and unjust.

Living now in Cadillac, Michigan, I left my house immediately after a phone call from my attorney informing me that my ex-husband would not be returning my children from visitation during spring break. I was informed he had enrolled them in school downstate. I must have been in shock because even now I remember extremely little about the one hundred and eighty-six mile panic-stricken drive down. I do remember however driving recklessly down a country dirt road, hysterically screaming, "I want to die!" toward the heavens.

As I approached a railroad track, I neither saw nor heard the train approaching until I was upon the tracks. The whistle blew frantically, I panicked slamming on the brakes, lost control of the car and spun around to a stop on the other side of the track facing the opposite direction. Dust was still clearing as the train whizzed on by on the tracks. Sobbing and shaking I don't know how long I sat there before I realized I was still alive and that it was by Grace of God and He had not answered my previous request to take my life.

Sometimes we do need to thank God for unanswered prayer! Instantaneously I realized God obviously had other plans for he had just spared my pitiful life after screaming at Him that I no longer wanted to live. I then set out on a life-long journey to discover exactly what those plans may be. That was over twenty-eight years ago. Notice what it took to change my direction, a near train wreck!

Many treasures following that immeasurable threatening incident have now been enlightened to my understanding. It was a *miracle* I was not killed that day! It made me stop and reflect on where I was, where I had been and where I was going. It opened my eyes to treasures unseen and the desire to begin a search for them. It simply was a miracle, a divine intervention of God to change my direction and turn me around, literally and spiritually. Just as it was when Paul raised the man from the dead who fell from the balcony at a meeting. Treasures in darkness often are overlooked unless we purpose to find them.

By this time my faith was finally beginning to increase while at the same time I was learning a deeper meaning of the scriptures, especially from James.

James 2:20-22. "You foolish man, do you want evidence that faith without deeds is useless? Was not our ancestor Abraham considered righteous for what he did when he offered his son Isaac on the altar? You see that his faith and his actions were working together and his faith was made complete by what he did "

His faith was made complete by what he did. We can say that we believe in anything, we trust anyone, but until we put *action* to the belief it is void. For example: I can write and/or speak the fact that I trust my physician with my life. When I do I can be sure in some manner or form a test of that declaration of faith will follow. In this instance the test of that profession of faith comes when I am told I am in need of surgical intervention. Perhaps I am told this is a very delicate procedure and along with it the possible risks of lifelong consequence. Sure, I can tell God and everyone else that I trust Him.

But, until I put action to that profession of faith and actually have the surgery it is invalid. Upon recovering from surgery successfully, then my faith in His abilities and my willingness to trust Him yet again increase. Faith like seeds, grows as it is watered.

God still parts Red Seas and miracles still happen today. Perhaps you are facing a questionable diagnosis of your own maybe with the possibility of a surgical intervention. Maybe it seems overwhelming and impossible, it feels as though it would take a miracle to overcome this one. A red-sea-parting may be needed. I believe in healing and I witnessed a miraculous healing. I never entertained the thought that I might be worthy of such a touch from our maker. That was for people of great faith and magnitude not someone like me. Then my closest friend and mentor was diagnosed with lung cancer.

Jeanette was a gracious friend, wonderful mom and the grandmother everyone wants to have. She taught me the value of leading others to Christ and she was not afraid to say to anyone, "Have you asked Jesus into your heart?" She loved her grandchildren with all her heart and brought them into her home for popcorn, videos and sleepovers many a week-end. I was amazed that as they grew into their teens they would give up time on a week-end with their friends to have that special time with grandma. I still strive today to model after her and I think of her dearly every time I hear wind chimes twinkling. She'd say listen an angel just flew by.

I spent many hours in prayer with her on the behalf of our families praying them through one situation after another and seeing many results. When Cancer invaded her life personally, believing in healing, many of us prayed for her. We fully expected to see the manifestation of that. However, she lost her battle with Cancer and it took me some time to reconcile with her death. I finally came to the conclusion that she *was* healed. Just not in the manner I or others desired, not according to our idea of healing. Initially I blamed Faith, mine, hers, and everyone else's. Until, revelation was exposed that healing comes in many forms.

I believe she is healed, in glory and probably still interceding for of all of us praising God and awaiting the day when she will once again share a very special time with her family and especially her beloved grandchildren. Red Seas are sometimes parted when the enemy advances, sometimes the power is bestowed for battle and sometimes the grace is given to endure the battle scars. Sometimes the prey is delivered from the battle.

I also witnessed a parting-of-the-seas following a seminar I had presented several years ago for wounded hearts. The focus at the time was mainly on victims of rape or incest and the plan was to offer hope to suffering individuals. This would then allow a forum in a trustworthy safe environment for individual victims to come forward and share their stories. It was April, a month designated for Sexual Assault Awareness and many of us were very busy gathering pamphlets, speakers and resources to promote such an event. Sara of whom you have become familiar in past chapters was designated to be the keynote speaker. This prompting others in our support group to come forward hesitantly but bravely to be part of the designated impact panel. An impact panel is a designated group of victims willing to share their feelings about victimization and the hope and victories following. It takes tremendous courage to come out of the shadows and share such intimate details so carefully hidden for so many years. Remember courage is not the lack of fear but rather the willingness to move forward in spite of fear and move forward they did!

The impact panel prepared and ready to present their stories even though anxious were very successful as was the first seminar in general. The sanctuary filled up with men and women ready to experience a new horizon. The room was buzzing with anticipation. The Keynote Speaker shared her story and then the Impact Panel was introduced. A Michigan State Police Officer, two local working housewives, and a youth minister. Three Incest Survivors, two female and one male and one female Domestic Violence Survivor shared openly and honestly their stories of humiliation and victim-ization; finally breaking years of silence.

Following the seminar, I received contact from two women who had attended. One of whom I previously knew but had no idea she had been a victim. I became aware that their memories and emotions had been stirred and were threatening to erupt like Mount Vesuvius in AD 79. Both made a decision to slam the door shut on the past and open the door of healing. It was as if the enemy were advancing from behind threatening to overtake them, the sea in front of them with what may have looked like no way out. However, the seminar offered a parting of the sea and a way of escape to the Promised Land. [Freedom]

For the following two years through support groups and individual counseling, I watched as these women both shared their pain, humiliation and subsequent healing! What appeared impossible was possible as emotionally and spiritually they advanced to the promise. From that seminar experience their identification with members of the panel helped them recognize that they were not alone in their victimization. They were not alone in their humiliation and they did not need to hide any longer. They recognized that in breaking the silence their was a freedom that led to significant changes in their lives. Miracles began as another sea was parted and how wonderfully exciting to witness such miracles in the lives of others.

Chapter Six

Breaking the Silence

This book has been dedicated to individuals who have suffered neglect and/or wounds of abuse; this chapter is dedicated to a young man whom I am not at liberty to name. However, I know I would have his approval to include this chapter. His name, circumstance and story has been altered *slightly* in order to protect family and all those connected with him. Any similarities to anyone you may recognize are purely coincidental.

It is designed to honor a man who identifies with some of the same torment you may have experienced. The wounds of grief and suffering pierced his heart deeply, so unfathomable and profound that the inconceivable came to pass. Running from the issues of his own heart, the appalling events of the past molded his character and consequently his behavior. It eventually forced him to become a man who was out of the bounds of rational control. The deafening cries from within his wounded heart prompted him to flee to a place where he could be alone with his brokenness. It is a place that led him nowhere except into deeper despair.

Some people come forward boldly and courageously telling their story to any and all who will listen, others cry silently in the night. Some of them wish to remain anonymous and others never get the chance to inform. I want to tell his story and I believe he would want me to.

What I remember most about this young man was the mocha-colored brown eyes that danced mischievously as he talked. His dark skin glistened in the light of the room as he anxiously began his story. Jeremiah, I will call him Jerry for short, walked anxiously into the room; a man with a mission. I made the usual attempts to solicit information and attempts at setting him at ease. He willingly complied and allowed me the opportunity to begin a trusting professional relationship.

He was not the first male I had counseled but certainly the first with such a unique situation. Following a phone call, he came that very day with a rather diverse purpose for initiating the session. He had not come for personal counseling but rather to seek guidance and develop an understanding of the patterns of abuse. Sexual abuse to be precise. The current love of his life had recently, as they became more physically intimate, developed a conscious surfacing of past memories of painful sexual incest in her life. This, he shared somewhat shyly, was affecting their intimate physical relationship. Because they were engaged and soon to be married he felt he needed to understand and support her. In fact, she herself was seeing a therapist. However she felt that it would be less embarrassing and healthier if he saw someone on his own.

We began to spend the time exploring materials and videos that were pertinent to her situation and his. He also spent time on his own exploring materials and researching the extremely complex subject of sexual incestuous relationships. I had in the past come across significant others with the very same purpose in mind. Two of them were parents and the other one a husband. Parents occasionally will seek advice to deal with a child who has been raped or discloses incest as well and I have had the pleasure to assist them in their quest for knowledge and information.

Somewhere in the weeks that followed, his eagerness to learn turned into frustration, anger and insomnia. As our sessions continued he openly shared that he was having nightmares along with bits and pieces of memory, called Flashbacks. This is typical of those who have repressed their memories of abuse. The flashes of memory were disturbing to him resulting in conflicting emotions and anger. Flashbacks are memories of past traumas. They may take the form of pictures, sounds, smells, body sensations, feelings or the lack of them (numbness). They may trigger a sense of panic, feeling spellbound and powerless with no memory stimulating it. These experiences may also occur in dreams. They are also a controversial subject in the professional world.

As explained previously, children {or adolescents} tend to insulate themselves from the emotional and physical horrors of trauma. In order to survive, the child may remain isolated, unable to express the feelings and thoughts of that time. The memory is put into a time capsule until it comes out full-scale into the present. When it does it is as if the experience in the past is now happening in the present. Intense sensations, both physical and mental may occur that are frightening. The victim begins to think they're mad or fanatical and fear telling anyone (including therapists) of these experiences. Sometimes as they surface the victim will attempt to push them back down unwilling to put the pieces together.

Through his determination however, Jerry was able to put some pieces together as he allowed the secrets locked deep with in him to finally surface. Through a project called diagramming he did what is called a timeline. Placing on a poster board a diagram of memories that were relative up to the current time. He sought verification from his father and other family as to the validity of the events he was beginning to recall. He discovered a long buried secret, he was not only the significant other he was a past victim of incest. A conflict began to develop between his desire to be supportive of his girlfriend and his own issues, but Jerry persevered including reaching out to other male victims. He desired to and finally did initiate a support group for African-American Male Victims. During this process, I felt however that he needed referral to additional sources that fit his therapeutic needs and he followed through with my suggestion willingly while still maintaining bi-monthly visits with me.

Oftentimes, victims fear the progression of moving forward to survival because of the emotional cost; feeling the pain is too high a price to pay. This however did not in the least dissuade him, he was willing to persevere. He explored his current level of faith and God became an intricate, indispensible part of his progression in recovery not that he did not question his faith at times as most of us in darkness often do.

A natural human response to trauma might be to attempt to cope with it in a way that excludes God. Sometimes causing us to take our lives into our own hands at the exclusion of His will for us. I believe however, that his faith carried him through the painful discoveries of the next two years. In attending sessions designed for him and with his fiancé, he faced a challenge that believers often do. He was required to superimpose the kingdom of God and those beliefs onto a system that is diametrically opposed to that order. In addition while still trying to gain the support of those that opposed him, he would angrily stomp around the counseling room and repeat again and again. "They just don't get it, Why don't they get it?" The frustration and agony was never more apparent than at those times.

As daunting a task as it was for him or would be for any *abused man* to undertake; the venue where we are called upon to do this, is the arena of our own wounded hearts. This is the residence of our wounds and the challenge to evict these memories is demoralizing especially with such little understanding and support of family or society. He bravely persevered regardless. He often spoke of many ways to develop community awareness and certainly could have been significant with his ordinary and bizarre ideas, however he lacked the confidence to initiate them. In his heart he wanted to share history, his story with the community which I hope I have done with justice. Unfortunately he is unable to take his story public now; the pain and darkness so overwhelming it lead him to a suicidal solution. It is our prayer that he rests in peace in the loving arms of the Savior who knows, who understands his pain.

If I could make one profound statement that I believe would be one that would come from his very lips: Listen to the little children, hear them, don't ignore their silent cries for justice and truth! In his journey to discovering his own abuse by an elder relative, a rage developed as he realized he was not listened to as a child. Currently, his family still refused to believe that his violations were anything more than young boys inappropriately experimenting as a result of raging hormones. Losing sight of his new found strength in Christ along with the humiliation at the hands of society, he became powerless to tolerate the ridicule and reality of his failure and thus took his life by the means suicide.

For centuries we have looked at Suicide as a demoralizing end to a devastating life. Suicide is often defined as the killing of one's self with malice aforethought, while in the possession of a sound mind {really?} How ironic? I would not say in such desperation and disillusionment that we are of sound mind. But that is my opinion. We search relentlessly for rational explanations and prevention. I believe fear, humiliation and hopelessness caused Jeremiah to give up on his quest to save children from the same violent victimization he had discovered as part of his past.

I continue the quest and I won't give up and as long as I have a voice. I will speak for Jeremiah and all the others who cannot. As long as I can, I will offer a forum for others who will break the silence. Fear is a crippling emotion that restrains a soul from moving forward. A binding emotion that alerts us when our very survival is threatened and then keeps the memories alive so we cannot function. There are times when fear surfaces for genuine, factual and authentic reasons and a sound mind is no longer sound.

Life's Shattered Pieces often lead to Fear and Fear to Isolation and hopelessness which often leads to Suicide. Picture with me a moment, you just sat down in your favorite comfy chair, a cold sweaty glass of ice tea in hand. The delicious aroma of lemon radiating from the top of the glass, a car door slams. You wonder who can that be? I'm not expecting anyone is your next thought as you glance out the window only to see two uniformed policemen advancing up the walk. By the grave look on their faces you immediately sense something is not good. Fear rises, a rush of adrenalin is released within your body, your heart races, your palms sweat and your knees get weak you get up to answer the door as the bell chimes.

Or, as you are matter-of-factly doing the Monday wash. You notice lipstick on the collar of your husband's shirt, not your shade you are thinking as the hair stands on end on your arms. Suddenly you feel an unusual knot in the pit of your stomach. You begin to tremble, Its fear!

The child victim of nightly incest may feel the same type of fear as soon as the creaking of the stairs begins the ascent of the perpetrator toward her bedroom door at the top. The knot in the stomach, the racing heart, the sweaty palms, the nausea. The tears begin as the handle on the doorknob turns, the dark shadow in the light of the hallway and the footsteps toward her bed. "No, not again she thinks as she hears the whispered voice." Shh! Don't cry, your mother will hear you and you know it would kill her." Fear rises within as she forces her self not to vomit and be quiet dreading what she knows is about to take place!

The woman above fears the officers have come to possibly present devastating news regarding a loved ones safety. The wife fears her husband may be having an affair and her marriage is about to end. The child fears another night of violation and physical abuse if she does not comply or the frightening consequence to her mother who has a serious heart condition. Intimidating crippling fear leaves an indelible devastating mark upon the soul. It may take years of perseverance and pain to remove it or at the very least become faded. It seems hopeless and many never try. Fear run wild cultivates discouragement, disillusionment and despair and for some overwhelming hopelessness.

We often believe that no one hears, no one knows, no one cares or understands and the result: Suicide! Our dear friend Jerry was unable to follow through, unable to turn it over, forgive himself and heal. His heart failed him. His intellect failed him and his memory failed him. Scripture states that hearts fail because of fear, how true.

2 Timothy 1:7 "For God hath not given us the spirit of fear; but of power and of love and of a sound mind. KJV

Shattered Pieces

Looking on the shattered pieces of my life
the broken torn places in my heart
like splintered glass, broken dreams, and strife
are my secrets from the dark.

Can I ever put them into place, the pieces of my past?
Will the pain ever cease, will meaning, vision or dream
ever come to pass?

"My child", said God. "Lay your heavy burdens down
the brokenness and pain.
All you need is mercy and grace
Your worry is ostensibly in vain."

I laid the pieces down.
Piece by shattered piece.
Gently He
made a way
Fashioning a Treasure beautiful into what I am today!

jtc "94"

Chapter Seven

Someone to Watch Over Me

Memories of past fear and abandonment for me take place in an upstairs old fashioned apartment building in the small rural Illinois town of Belvidere. The apartment was small, the stairway wooden with rubber mats in the middle, I suppose to deter slipping. The smell was a mixture of several resident's cooking and a mustiness I will never forget. The kitchen had a small dining ell that was designed to house a table and chairs for eating with a rounded arch dividing it from the food preparation area. That dining ell was my makeshift bedroom that contained what they used to call in those days, a roll-away-bed and a night stand. I had a scenic view of the kitchen sink and a garbage can that sat near the entrance to the bathroom. It was an eerie room because the ceilings were very high and in the bathroom a glass skylight above. I always feared someone was watching me. The only light however in the room shimmered from that skylight on a clear moonlit night. I was alone, which was not unusual as my mother and step-father made frequent trips to the local bars for recreation.

I remember those nights alone, even though I was very young, around six or seven. They would lock the door, warning me never to answer or open it to anyone, even if I knew or thought I knew them. I would clutch closely to my chest my little tiny tears doll as large crocodile tears streamed down my face. I don't know what was more terrifying, the sound of the creaking stairs as footsteps could be heard occasionally in the hall, or the sight of cockroaches scampering about the garbage for their nightly meal.

My mother wasn't deliberately negligent, she simply had to choose between my alcoholic stepfather and me. She chose him, so typical of a dysfunctional domestically-violent home. I understand now as knowledge and experience has revealed, the difficulty for the co-dependent [significant other] trying to keep a dysfunctional home functional. Fortunately for me, I had reprieve from that home through sporadic times of visiting with my grandparents. Good times, times of peace, security and love. Most importantly faith! I had someone to watch over me, though at the time, I might not have understood the breadth and depth of such an assignment.

My stepfather was a character when he was sober and my love for country music came from Sundays in the park with him. I would sit listening to a transistor radio [for the younger crowd these were definitely not like an IPod]. I listened and learned to love music and nature. He drank and fished in the creek. Occasionally, I would wander off in exploration. In those days it was safe and I would work up enough courage to cross the catwalk [a swinging bridge] over the creek. Until, he would come to find me, scold me for taking off and interrupting his fishing and swing the bridge till I would scream for mercy. Those time were good times but few and far between the intoxications, and the yelling and violence that resulted. I developed a pattern of fear along with expectations that good times never last, because they never did.

I lived anxiously awaiting the next crisis, as most of you do who live in abusive situations or alcoholic homes. You know the fear and anxiety that promotes a sickening deep-gut feeling that something insurmountable, uncontrollable is about to happen. You know it, you recognize it, you've felt it. Your heart begins to race, your palms sweat, your stomach tightens with that queasy feeling. The tears well up, but you choke them back. You try to convince yourself you are just acting crazy, being ridiculous. But you sense the unknown is about to make its untimely appearance once again into your life, molding, crippling, shaping a pattern of chaos that would take a lifetime to disengage.

Fortunately, *someone* was watching over me and it was not just my loving grandparents. My lonely fear-filled nights would come to an abrupt end in a sudden and hurried courtroom drama. A man behind a huge mahogany desk in a black robe would send me this time to live permanently with my grandparents in Michigan. Finally! Finally I would be safe, cared for, loved, clothed and fed. My emotional, physical and spiritual needs met. I was introduced to an entity far above all that I could possibly imagine. Today, I would tell you that a power greater than any on Earth had control of my life and its' destiny. It would prove itself over the years to be of a magnitude beyond belief and exceedingly more than I could imagine. It is obvious as I look back over the roller coaster moments of my life that this power was in control along with a plan for keeping me safe.

Jeremiah 1:5 "Before I formed you in the womb I knew you, before you were born I set you apart; I appointed you as a prophet to the nations" and Jeremiah 29:11 "For I know the plans I have for you", declares the Lord, "plans to give you a hope and a future"

As I may have said before, Treasures hidden in darkness are not often seen in the natural, they sometimes take supernatural faith, supernatural spiritual-vision. We may not visualize at first, divine revelation. We may need seeking him, asking him, listening for him and then moving forward. It was a divine intervention that moved me from a turbulent situation and calmed the stormy seas. Someone was watching over me!

It was a miracle when Jesus walked on water and when the storm was silenced by His very word. *Matthew 8:26 "And he saith unto them, Why are ye fearful, O ye of little faith? The he arose and rebuked the winds and the sea; and there was a great calm. KJV*

I have always been taught that Faith is the evidence of things not seen. Actually calling forth things that are not as though they were. We often need to do just that; we may just need to dig a ditch! Not literally of course. A spiritual ditch. Say you were a farmer in desperate need of more water on your land. Your current well run dry. If you were actually in need of water calling forth a miracle of God to provide it, believing that he will; then you may need to put action with your vision. In other words, taking the step to dig a ditch and expecting Him to fill it.

There may even be times when you may need to take a greater step of Faith and walk on water; so to speak! Picture it, my well has run dry, my farm is suffering, my animals becoming dehydrated. "Lord, I speak water onto this land!" I have called forth what is not as though it were. Now it is time for me to dig an additional well and thank God that He will fill it. But, if I want to move with great Faith as in the proverbial "walking on water", I will not only dig the ditch but buy more cattle. Our steps may be into unknown territory and we may need to act with no real assurance or response and *wait* for results. Wait!

Chapter Eight

Waiting for Miracles

Treasures may be found during the waiting for miracles as well as in receiving them. Sometimes waiting for your miracle may perhaps be as difficult as believing for one. In these days and times we all seem to want instant gratification. We want what we want when we want it. Usually that is yesterday. We often think we are unique; the only one who has come up against barriers to our goals. But taking a look at the Israelites as they trusted in their leader, Moses, to deliver them out of the hands of the Egyptians, notice the spirit of doubt and unbelief that existed even in that time.

Go back with me in time. The Israelites are ready to begin a long journey, their destiny has been foretold. In my imagination they are anxious to get going leaving the horrors of the past behind, hopeful for the future and they are motivated! It must have taken tremendous Faith, determination and preparation as they left their present lifestyle. As uncomfortable as it was, they were accustomed to difficulty. Anything would be better than being stuck in bondage to slavery. They had hope, and they had a vision of what had been foretold. A promise of provision, freedom and unseen treasures.

Scripture tells us they experienced supernatural episodes along the way, however impatient and wallowing in unbelief cost some of them fulfillment of their destiny. They begun their journey as we often do with enthusiasm and passion. They had vision and a plan of action. However, the first time they encounter a major obstacle [The

Red Sea], they complain and question. Imagine Moses, all the complaints are directed at him; the once esteemed leader now becomes the scapegoat for their dilemma.

I can relate, can you? Have you ever trusted in something or someone to help you reach your destination and suddenly plans were disrupted? Disappointed we may tend to project the blame on a colleague if it is work related or a partner if home related. Husbands and wives, brothers and sisters are notorious for doing this.

Here, Moses in obedience to the request of God had followed the chosen path and now he was the scapegoat for the Israelites anger and disappointment. There must have appeared to be no way out. Impatience and most likely fear becomes their focus. They couldn't turn back they would've been captured and returned to a more devastating captivity than beforehand. The massive obstacle in front of them must have seemed overwhelmingly impossible to overcome. There was no outlet to the right or left and no alternative but to stand still. Good point, worth repeating. When you can't move forward nor go back, when there is no outlet to the right or left. Stand still!

Exodus 14:13 "Stand firm and you will see the deliverance the Lord will bring you today." NIV

Isaiah 40:31 "But they that wait upon the Lord, shall renew their strength, they shall mount up with wings as Eagles, they shall run and not be weary, they shall walk and not faint."

If your patience is anything like mine, then you hate waiting for anything. Whether it is in a grocery line or waiting for anticipated mail or phone calls; it all seems like a waste of time. I want what I want, and I want it yesterday. I even fold laundry while I am waiting for the computer to load, wash dishes while on the phone. Fortunately, their leader, Moses was not as impatient and not moved by the crowd's demands. He stood his ground, drew upon his Faith. He called out in belief to God putting into "action" that Faith. God honored and answered and gave specific instruction. They advanced and as they did, then the sea parted {the obstacle moved out of the way as they moved forward in Faith believing}. The enemy followed but was destroyed and they were safe! A sea parted...a miracle! They waited, they received, Faith strengthened! Note that Faith and action moves obstacles out of the way.

Isaiah 40:31 "But they that wait upon the Lord shall renew their strength"

Undoubtedly, you have never witnessed a literal parting of a sea. But maybe like me, you have had situations that appeared hopeless and impossible and those situations changed as you moved forward in spite of them. An abused wife feels trapped in her situation. She ponders the thoughts: "If I stay I will continue to be physically hurt. If I leave how will I support myself, where will I stay and will he come after me?" Finally, the situation becomes so desperate that she may have to leave suddenly nor have time to make some preparation. The situation feels hopeless as she leaves. She cannot move forward there appears to be no solution, she can't go back now fearing the abuse will intensify. Those of you who have been there know that it does intensify. She doesn't have the money to obtain shelter. She doesn't want to impose on others. I was in that situation once and fortunately as I sought God for an answer the professionals led me to a shelter and many doors opened for relief. I could not go back the only way to go was forward in Faith and allow God to move the obstacles.

The treasure in that darkness, I was learning God could be trusted and would make a way where there seemed to be none. It also was the beginning of breaking-the-silence of my violent victimization of the past as they offered a safe forum to share those incidents. A very dark sea parted and treasure began to unfold!

Chapter Nine

Buried Treasure

Treasures are often within reach but obscured by our own desires or actions. Are you yet convinced that miracles do happen; Divine supernatural interventions of God in your life? If so I applaud you. Read on to discover your riches [hidden] in secret places. If you are still pondering or among the doubters read on anyway!

If God actually parted an entire Sea for escape from your difficulties would you then believe? Most likely. Does He still part seas today? Metaphorically speaking, yes! As Paul Harvey, a famous radio commentator used to say, "Now for the rest of the story". Whew! They're safe! God rolled back the waters for the Israelites and destroyed the enemy advancing upon them. No sooner are they saved from destruction however, than they began to murmur and complain in fear of provision.

Exodus 15:24 "And the people murmured against Moses saying, What shall we drink?" KJV

They saw none of the promises, where was this promised land flowing with provision? They again turned on their deliverer. You can almost hear them saying, "This is a fine mess you've got us into Moses, nothing to eat or drink. It's hot and how are we going to survive? We were better off in Egypt at least we had food and drink." How quickly they've forgotten!

About now you may be criticizing them with questions like: How could they possibly forget the miracle they just received? Didn't God just part a sea for them? I used to do the same thing. I would wonder how they could have acted that way. What an attitude! Then I realized I have, at times, demonstrated the same approach. A disappointment, a lost job or failed relationship may turn us toward or away from God. If we ask for help, for circumstances to improve, they do and we are ever so thankful. Praising God for moving the mountains, parting our seas. However, time passes and another challenge presents itself. We feel the anxiety threatening to overwhelm us and things are not changing quickly enough, discouragement sets in. We focus on the problem and not the problem-solver. Suddenly, we forget where our previous help came from.

Psalm 121:1-2 "Where does my help come from? My help comes from the LORD." NIV

If God was able to part an *entire* sea for the Israelites, could he not undoubtedly provide food? We hinder His miracle-working power with our lack of gratitude, just as the Israelites did. Hopefully, we will not have to wander in the wilderness for forty years as they did to recognize His power. There were treasures to be found in their darkness, riches hidden in secret places but they failed to believe, so they failed to find. Let's look at the treasures and the Israelites hindrances to discovering them. Take some time to explore Exodus in scripture as to just how close they were to their desired promise and missed it!

Have you got any rivers to cross, any mountains too big to climb? Some days it would seem so. One day we are moving along hungrily with anticipation, suddenly around the corner appears a massive boulder in the way of our progress. It must have seemed that way after the Israelites crossed the sea and were now fearing for food to survive. They remembered the sweltering breath of the enemy hot on their trail and their emotions began to waver, just as ours do. When Lord? Where Lord, How Lord? Are we there yet? Sounds like the whining of a child doesn't it? Our limited vision unfortunately only allows us to see the huge boulder threatening to obstruct our progress. Feeling overwhelmed, too many issues, not enough time, not enough energy, and not enough money. Not enough, not enough, not enough! But, God is absolutely more than enough. Through scripture Paul assures us that in times of need God is more than enough, In times of weariness, He will provide the rest needed.

Philippians 4:19 "But my God shall supply all your need according to his riches in glory by Christ Jesus" KJV

He will provide to those that come, rest to the weary and heavy-laden.

Matthew ll:28 "Come unto me, all ye that labour and are heavy laden, and I will give you rest." Matthew 17:20 "If you have faith as small as a mustard seed, you can say to this mountain, 'Move from here to there and it will move'. Nothing will be impossible for you."

Were the treasures of darkness in the Red Sea and wilderness Israelite experience buried? Let's look for a moment at some of the treasures.

Treasure is not always buried.......

THE TREASURES [From The Exodus]

1. The Israelites learned to extend their Faith as they left behind all they were accustomed to; in order to follow their esteemed leader, Moses
2. They were freed from bondage to slavery.
3. They found camaraderie as they united together in their common cause.
4. God fulfilled His promise of provision [provided manna]
5. God provided safety.
6. God removed their greatest obstacle [The Sea] from their path.
7. God delivered them from their oppressors.

I believe if we continued to investigate further we would discover more treasures. As the story unfolds the Israelites failed to focus on the treasure from heaven but rather on their current circumstance or challenges. As *we* often do. What were the obstacles [hindrances] that altered that focus? I believe it was the following:

HINDRANCES [of the Israelites]

1. Lack of Gratitude
2. Fear
3. Doubt
4. Unrealistic Expectations
5. Disobedience
6. Anger
7. Unforgiveness
8. Criticism/Complaint

Just like the Israelites we often miss the treasures in dark places due to unrealistic expectations. We attempt to put God in a box made of our specifications. We lose sight of our vision and His promises. We allow distractions to dissuade and hinder our progress. But, all hope is not lost! If we are willing to gain knowledge of the things that stand in our way, crucify self then with God's help we will be able overcome those things that so easily beset us.

Hebrews 12:1 "let us lay aside every weight, and the sin which doth so easily beset us, and let us run with patience the race that is set before us." KJV

Chapter Ten

Crossing Our Red Sea

D o you know that a heart of gratitude opens our eyes of under-standing so as to distinguish the treasures that lie in the dark-ness? Gratitude is remembering the wonderful things that others have done for us with a attitude of thankfulness. Most of us do nice things for each other without expectation of a return, however it feels amazing to know the act of kindness is appreciated. God is not different though loving and kind; He also desires to know that His acts of kindness toward us are appreciated.

Have you ever had a friend who has helped you time and time again giving their energy, time or maybe even sacrificed to help you? If you never showed appreciation, never thanked them, never acknowledged their sacrifice; how long do you think they would remain a friend or at the very least continue to help you? If worse than that you complained about what was given, murmuring and criticizing; do you think they would continue to give? Lack of grati-tude can hinder our focus rather than enabling us to see value in what we have received. We miss the treasure!

The fear of the Israelites hindered them and a heart of fear hin-ders us from taking the necessary steps to discover God's hidden treasure. "Phobos" for which the word phobia comes, means "flight" or that which may cause flight. Synonyms include; cowardice, terror, dread, or panic. You finally have a dream or desire to do something extraordinary. You're energized, planning and preparing, thinking about it day and night. Then suddenly out of some unknown place within, you become panicky. Little doubts creep into the recesses of your mind. You begin to question your motives and your abilities. The motivation begins to fade and your thoughts become failure orientated. Fear becomes irrational and your vision is now blinded. No longer can we see the treasure and now doubt that it will ever come to pass. The result? Missed opportunity.

2 Timothy 1:7 "For God hath not given us the spirit of fear; but of power, and of love, and of a sound mind." KJV

I learned that if I don't believe treasure exists in darkness [or dark circumstances] I won't look for it. If I don't look for it, I may not find it! Lack of Faith while hindering motivation also hinders trust. I have had circumstances where my lack of trust that the vision could actually materialize cost me years of delay. By the way delay is not always denial.

In addition, I have allowed in the past a "lack of trust" or belief that my circumstance would ever end to cause me much unneeded anxiety. Fear nullifies Faith. Scripture tells us without Faith it is impossible to please God, after all it is Faith that moves the hand of God. If fear nullifies Faith, Faith moves God and without Faith I cannot please God; then Fear will keep God from moving in my circumstance and not please Him. Delay and anxiety with lack of result, therefore; Faith is what I needed.

I got tired of prolonging painful circumstances or hindering His promises because of my unbelief. With God all things are possible if we will believe, well maybe not all but certainly those which He has preordained or purposed for our lives. It only takes one step, one single step forward to begin a journey!

Humanity, of course, in this day and age demands proof. Faith is believing without proof. So it goes against everything we have experienced thus far and no wonder it is such a difficult task for some. I have however, an example, that demonstrates that I had finally come to a place in my life where tiny mustard seed Faith was developing. Unseen and unfortunate circumstances had forced me into a diminishing financial situation. I was on a mudslide, downhill all the way and my entire future was threatened. All my resources were coming to an end and I was once again crying out to God for a miracle. Not only had I lost my car due to a head-on collision, was physically injured and off work but devastating changes at work were commencing.

Surely I could figure a way out of this mess, notice the I in that sentence? Initially I felt fear but following earnest prayer, God directed me to utilize my skills and make a list of goals, objectives, obstacles and possible solutions. In so doing, it became apparent that selling my home was the obvious solution, thereby downsizing my current expenses. Sounds easy right? Not so much! We were in a statewide downward real estate spiral. Nothing was selling quickly [and still isn't]. I was willing to follow through with what I felt God was leading me to do, but He would have to sell my home. Obviously, I needed a miracle. I stood in Faith, I claimed to everyone who would listen that I was trusting God to sell my condo. I did not put it on the market but I did hold a weekend open house on my own that brought two lookers but no sale.

The following Wednesday in church, I gave a simple verbal prayer request that led to the sale of that home. A man who visited our church infrequently just happened [?] to be looking for a condo in our area. He approached me after the service and immediately came to look at it. There were a few tests along the way of my self-declaration of Faith that God would do this but eventually the sale was completed. A miracle had taken place.

You may believe it was coincidence [what is coincidence anyway?]. I believe it was divine intervention. A miracle! Restoration had taken place, the buyer was restored spiritually in the process, my bank account financially! Several comparable condos in that same complex listed for considerably less money, on the market for up to three years and mine sold in a few weeks for thousands of dollars more.

Just a side note, I put a sign out front afterwards, "God Sold Mine" The treasure in darkness? My prayers were answered, my finances restored and *my faith* strengthened. Subsequent to the sale, I was exhilarated. Nothing could stop me now, after all, God was on my side. I moved ahead ready to conquer the world feeling indestructible and as though I could accomplish anything. Ready to run the race set before me.

Chapter Eleven

The Tortoise and The Mare

No, that is not a typographical error. It is meant to say Mare, not Hare. You may be reflecting on Aesop's Fable, "The Tortoise And The Hare" at this very moment, but my story is rearranged a bit. If you recall, the hare or rabbit in Aesop's Fable was eager to win the race, confidently running ahead then repeatedly backtracking to discover what might be holding up his counter part, the tortoise. At one point so over-confident that he loses his focus on the finish line and lies down under a tree to take a nap. His pride and idleness, of course cost him the victory. It was a missed opportunity to say the least. Remember the tortoise almost lifeless and unhurried just saunters along taking his time ever so slowly. His journey calculated and deliberate and never wavering in his purpose. Conserving his energy, never losing focus, his goal in sight.

Like the tortoise some of us begin passively when it comes to reaching out to receive our miracles or complete our destiny. We experience a vision or a desire begins to burn in our heart undoubtedly from God and we become excited at first. Many times the passion eventually fizzles out. The timings not right, the children are still in school, insufficient funding or maybe when the kids are out of college. Then finally, I'm too old now! It never comes to pass, the dream aborted.

Why the change in my story from Hare to Mare? There are those of us that fit neither original category, beginning the race passively as the tortoise or with overwhelming energy as the hare losing sight of the goal by constantly backtracking. We would better be described as a mare. Untamed, wild and full of exuberance. Give us the plan and purpose and we are off and running. Full of passion and like a racehorse we bolt out of the starting gate as the bell rings. In full gallop we run ahead before we know who, what, where, when, and especially how we are going to accomplish the goal and finish the race.

A good start certainly helps to win a race but equally of value is that last stretch before the finish line, If we exhaust all resources at the launch, we will have none left for the finale. Without a doubt sometimes giving up frustrated as obstacles emerge. We need moderation, balance, a trainer, something or someone pulling back our reins. And in our case it never pays to run ahead of God.

Like, the Israelites we now see we experience the lack of gratitude, fear, doubt, and unrealistic expectations. We still need to explore the final three hindrances to obtaining our miracles, completing the journey to our promise. Anger. Righteous indignation or unrighteous retaliation? Indignation has its' place and time surfacing when we witness or experience acts of injustice. Anger for a cause, if you will? We believe and sometimes rightly so that our anger is justified. How we cope with and express it may or may not be appropriate. Anger can be detrimental to us in several ways, some of which we may have addressed but lets refresh ourselves for a moment.

From incapacitating blinding migraines to ulcers, hypertension and irritable bowels we note that internalized anger entertained on a sustained basis is extremely detrimental to our physical being. Unfortunately, the only treasure I see in the above is in the bank accounts of physicians. Depression [anger turned inward] is also definitely destructive to our spiritual and emotional well-being as well. No one actually makes us angry. We choose or choose not to be. Situations may occur which result in angry feelings but thoughtful consideration and communication most often can diffuse a potentially volatile state of affairs. However, once sufficient time has been taken to review a situation action should then be imminent. Otherwise, if allowed to brew we become overly aggressive or combative.

Choosing to be angry or not, may require a power greater than ourselves to assist in the matters of extreme anger where violation has occurred, surely your spouse forgetting to take your best suit to the cleaners is not as serious as a rape or physical violation. There is however, no justification for out-of-control anger when the God who controls all things has given us His Spirit, a treasure within to assist us with self-control, a most critical point in this stage of removing hindrance to your destination. Perhaps you have struggled in this area on occasion or your lifetime. If you have not experienced the power of the Holy Spirit, now would be an opportune time to search out such a precious divine gift, yours for the asking. [I Corinthians 12] Ask God for supernatural power, one fruit of the Spirit is self-control. Believing in miracles for yourself takes Faith. Faith cometh by hearing and hearing by the word of God.

Miracles had begun to take place in my life strengthening my belief and I was witnessing them in the lives of others. There are times when we need to *look* for the treasures in darkness and times when we may need to *listen*. Keeping our spiritual eyes and ears open may be vital to recognition of them. It was a miracle when Peter and John healed the leper at the gate and a miracle when a church friend diagnosed with a tumor of her left breast. She went through the usual medical preliminaries, as we all stood with our faith believing that she would be healed. She was admitted to the hospital for a lumpectomy and possible mastectomy. Her husband took a stand of faith and declared healing for his wife. She was prepped, medicated and ready for surgery. She was under the influence of the medication and very groggy when the surgeon came in to explain that they would take one more x-ray prior to excision of the tumor.

They wheeled her down and x-rayed her left breast where a previous mammogram had shown the lump to be. Later after returning to her room he questioned her regarding the lump, verifying that it was indeed the left side. He then stated he wanted to x-ray the right breast as they had found no lump on the left.

She simply informed him she knew exactly which side the lump had been on and no they were not going to x-ray the right side, she was going home. Can you imagine how indignant you would feel someone trying to tell you after weeks of testing, mammograms where your lump is when you are the one who discovered it in the first place? She recognized that her prayer was answered. She was healed and still groggy left for home with her husband. That was several years ago and the lump has not returned, it was a healing miracle. Faith without works is dead and sometimes we just need to put our feet where our mouth is. Of course, I am not meaning to put your foot in your mouth though I have several times. Simply put: don't just talk the talk, walk it!

Treasures hidden in the darkness are not often seen in the natural, they sometimes take supernatural insight. We may not at first visualize them we may need revelation, we may have to ask, listen and then move! The important point here is to believe it, speak it and then do it! You will find that it takes action to bring it to pass. Turn that little Faith into Great Faith and miracles will come to pass. Just as it was a miracle when Jesus walked on water and when the storm was silenced by His word.

Matthew 8:26 [from the King James Version]says; "And he saith unto them, Why are ye fearful, O ye of little faith? Then He arose, and rebuked the winds and the sea; and there was a great calm."

Chapter Twelve

Don't Let The Sun Go Down
On Your Wrath

W e have established anger as one of the obstacles for the Israelites and it can be an obstacle to recovery for the abused. Stored Anger breeds Unforgiveness. Have you ever be so unjustifiably hurt that you thought you would never be able to get over it? People or circumstances may have devastated you, but with help you can respond in forgiveness, some circumstances just take longer than others and powers greater than ourselves.

We want to experience an abundant life; rich and full of all that we were destined to have and be. But unresolved anger, unending rage and resentment is definitely a spiritual blockade to receiving all God has designed for us. It is definitely a barrier or hindrance to our inheritance as a child of God. Remember you are not a victim of your circumstance unless you choose to be. Remember our motto. "Do not let the past determine who you are; rather who you become!"

Devastating circumstances are obviously more complex and difficult to overcome, sometimes overwhelming to say the least. Where there is willingness, there is a way. A well respected author and friend, Pastor Edwin Murray once told a story at an evening service he was teaching with regard to motivation when overcoming obstacles. It goes something like this, [emphasis mine].

Picture a warm breezy afternoon, you just happen to stroll into the yard and notice a stray cat desperately trying to out run a pack of wild dogs. You glance behind the cat and notice a Rottweiler, Doberman Pincher and Pit Bull in hot pursuit of the poor feline. Would you intervene and risk possible severe injury to save the cat? Probably not, the risks outweigh the benefit, the obstacles appear overwhelming and success almost impossible. Unless of course you are a cat lover [I am] and extremely courageous [I am not]. I don't believe I could take on three dogs of that caliber.

Suppose the circumstances were a tad different. The wild dogs appear angry, foaming at the mouth and vicious, but instead of pursuit of the cat, they are approaching attack of your child playing innocently in the yard. Circumstances have changed, motivation has changed and obstacles are of no concern at the moment. You will risk your life to save the life of your child regardless!

The potential is directly proportionate to the motivation. The same application may be made in any situation. This contests all pretexts we make against forgiveness and eradicates the word impossible. Our ability to forgive in any circumstance is directly proportionate to the motivation to do so. In some cases of severe abusiveness and violation it may however take a divine intervention to assist us. Our only responsibility is to be willing and in extreme complexities we may need to initially begin with a willingness to be willing. If you are holding resentment, Unforgiveness or offense in your heart, now would be an ideal time to ask divine help to eradicate it.

If this is unfamiliar territory for you explore it slowly and with a guide. For most of us traveling this journey it is one road at a time. The unknown may occasionally present an unexpected detour with a DANGER sign warning us of impending hazard. One of the most significant detours on the journey to freedom and ultimately our destiny is unresolved anger. I am not referring to minor frustration, such as with a child, spouse or friend, but rather bondage to repressed resentful irate emotion. Rape, murder or personal violation of any sort is a catalyst of this type of anger to the utmost degree. Reaching a place of letting go, forgiving takes a great deal of persevering effort.

Anger wears many diverse disguises and is perhaps the most destructive of all emotion. The full reason I spend so much energy addressing it. Unrestrained it is the foundation for external acts of violence and internal roots of bitterness. *Ephesians 4:26 "Be angry, and yet do not sin"* Scripture teaches us to not let the Sun go down on our wrath. No matter what degree your anger may have reached, you can take steps to obliterate its' evil toxin. Instead make it work for you in a positive manner turning it into peace.

There are many degrees of the emotion, anger and the most destructive and explosive is rage; a vicious desire to retaliate or destroy someone or something in a verbal or physical manner. If you are a member of the abused population, you most likely have found yourself in the sudden grip of rage. Take a moment, reflect upon how you dealt with that rage, the consequence to you or others and how you felt afterward. How might it be different were you in a similar situation today, if that were to occur?

A more common and less severe form of anger could be described as a seething inner turmoil. Possibly brought about by an unjust situation or offense perpetrated against you or a loved one. The anger is turned inward [suppressed] causing turmoil emotionally and possibly physical manifestation such as eating disorders or addiction. There are healthy ways to cope with anger and release suppressed anger, however let's look at one more type of anger first.

The power of thinking positive for as a man thinketh in his heart so is he is paraphrased from sayings we have heard repeated over and over in our lifetime. Pastor Jim, my shepherd for many years always uses one of his favorites frequently, "Complain and Remain, Praise and Be Raised". Finding those treasures in darkness will never materialize for the complainer.

We would do well to reflect upon the Israelites again. All they had been delivered from, released from slavery. They were given the promise of provision and received it, protection and received it, they witnessed miracles. Yet when their individual expectations did not materialize they began to complain. The end result, to stay behind in the desert for the remainder of their lifetime. That entire generation did not see the promise land wandering in the wilderness [wastelands] for forty years, yet the promise was so close by. To put it simply, their desire for instant gratification was extinguished by God with a lesson of longsuffering and patience. I prefer to learn from their experience and not wander forty years in the wilderness, how about you?

I wish I could say there have never been times in my life when I complained or criticized the way God worked things out. Unfortunately, I have. Maybe not directly, but definitely indirectly. When we question what is happening or ask, Why? Is that not criticism, is it not complaint? Does it not show our creator that we question His decision for our better good? After all, if we accepted His decision, really accepted it, we would do it joyfully with thanksgiving, wouldn't we?

My oldest granddaughter was fifteen and approaching one of the most significant passages in a teenager's life. The moving from dependence upon others for transportation to the maneuvering of an automobile on her own. Yes, the infamous driving an automobile! She was to begin Driver's Education at school the following Monday and bubbled over with anticipation with one exception. She had never been behind the wheel of a car. With an impish twinkle in my eye, I politely told her how excited I was that she had reached this plateau in her teenage life; that on Monday I would be sure to be off the road and on my knees! She did not find that as amusing as I did.

Apparently, other students and friends of hers had driving time in an automobile and that opportunity for Ashleigh had not presented itself. Due to circumstances, no one else was available to provide driving experience prior to her class but Grandma. Now mind you, it had been several years since teaching my daughters to drive. We proceeded to the Church parking lot and a nervous teen moved into the driver's seat of my new car! Little did she realize that her first lesson would focus on fundamentals, not on the actual driving of the car. We went through road safety guidelines, turning on the key, hand placement, braking and adjusting mirrors. We both survived.

I tell you all that to make the point, had she complained or criticized the fact that she was only allowed to experience the basics, I most likely would have been hesitant to take her out for repeat lessons. She was not only cheerful and grateful but also permeable to anything she was taught or experienced, which stirred my desire to give her even more. I believe that is also the image of God's desire to bestow upon us. As we are thankful to him for the circumstance we are in? If so, He will lead us into better situations. So complain and remain, or praise and be raised!

A simple request in Faith to a loving Father who desires to give us so much more than we can imagine is all that is needed to illuminate the treasure in the midst of darkness. Don't let the Sun go down on your wrath, give it to the one who knows what to do with it and show you the way through it. Joy cometh in the morning!

Chapter Thirteen

Acquiring Treasure

In the past chapters we have taken a look at digging into the painful circumstances of the past to hunt for treasure, riches, destiny, and methods of turning obstacles into opportunities. Discovering in the process several ways of accomplishing that; but we can also just acquire treasures. One of the definitions of acquire is to obtain, get a hold of, or gain. Unlike something that takes energy as in searching or digging for.

In the process of writing this book the past few years, I have gained the ultimate revelation of the promise of *Isaiah 45:3 "I will give you the treasures of darkness; riches stored in secret places, so that you may know..."* I have known *about* Jesus from childhood, I have learned *of* Jesus through the adult years. I have developed a *relationship* with Him as a Christian in that progression from age five to this day as a senior. However, the revelation of His undying love, unfailing provision, longsuffering patience, abundant mercy and grace has never been more apparent than in the latest trial of my Faith.

I know He is, as He said He was, "I AM". It is as if He is standing there saying: "Do you need strength? I AM. Do you need light in the darkness, I AM. Do you need [anything]? I AM!" He is a swift arrow of light to the world of darkness. I personally will not be broken, my Spirit refuses to be crushed by circumstance, my failures or the enemy. Continued adversity has served to rise within me a rebel streak to fight, to win, to live. I will hide in His quiver all the days of my life so that He will be glorified! I thank God for the Hope that is now within me. I thank God for Salvation, a free gift to you and me there for the choosing. A treasure in the darkness of life simply waiting to be discovered and acquired by all.

If at this point you do not know Jesus, have not asked Him to live within you. Today may be just the day to make that confession by Faith, today may be the day for you to receive a miracle, the miracle of rebirth. If you are ready, my prayers are with you as you make the confession following. If not, the treasure is here for you to acquire whenever you are ready to receive it.

ABC's

I <u>Accept</u> and <u>Acknowledge</u> that Jesus died for my sin and I repent from all sin and wrongdoing in my life as He brings them to my remembrance, I <u>Believe</u> that He is and ever shall be and that belief on the Lord Jesus Christ brings me and my household salvation and I <u>Confess</u> the Lord Jesus Christ as my Savior!

"But God commendeth his love toward us, in that, while we were yet sinners, Christ died for us" (Romans 5:8).KJV

"But your iniquities have separated between you and your God, and your sins have hid his face from you, that he will not hear" (Isaiah 59:2).KJV

"That if thou shalt confess with thy mouth the Lord Jesus, and shalt believe in thine heart that God hath raised him from the dead, thou shalt be saved" (Romans 10:9).KJV

Part Two

Riches Hidden In Secret Places

Chapter One

In The Darkest Places

In my search to discover God's hidden treasures in the midst of life circumstances, I have discovered as you have now witnessed, blessings. Blessings I was not often aware of at the time but never-the-less proved to be blessings just the same. In God's merciful unconditional love there has always been a blessing somewhere though hidden at times.

Picture yourself aboard a ship that has sailed through many rough seas and weather-beaten storms; carrying a cargo entrusted to you by God. A ship so enormous you would be most likely unable to maneuver if placed at the helm. Be calm dear soul, God is the Master. He has control and He has no intention of allowing you to sink. Your journey is safe with Him even as the storm arises.

A ship with a wise shipmaster on a voyage carries only the cargo needed to fulfill its consignment. How foolish then, to carry the overwhelming weight of past sails, unclaimed goods, or damaged shipments. Thus only weighing down the ship, slowing down the journey and possibly jeopardizing a safe arrival to its destiny. Yet, in the Soul or Spiritual Life, man tends to do these things. He may carry the burdens of Unforgiveness, resentment and pain of the past into the present. The burden in some cases becomes overwhelming and threatening to the entire existence therefore blinding the vision to the riches God has in store for us.

Isaiah 43:18 "Remember ye not the former things, consider ye not the things of old." and our key scripture: Isaiah 45:3 "I will give you the treasures of darkness; riches stored in secret places, so that you may know that I am the LORD, the God of Israel, who summons you by name" NIV.

The God of Israel, who summons you by name will show you the hidden riches so that you may know that he is Lord! He *is* the ruler over all things! He is sovereign over prosperity and adversity; both needed for us to grow spiritually and in character. His grace and mercy however are sufficient as the experience prepares us for destiny and eternity.

Think about this for a moment. What is the dark night of the Soul? How dark is dark? Dim, shadowy, murky, ominous? Even in the darkest of the dark, in the deepest depths there are hidden riches. Though difficult to clearly see at the time; looking back brings the realization of riches, great riches, if only in the fact that our loving Savior was carrying us through those times.

A marriage of sixteen years ends, custody battles ensue, lives and their direction are changed forever. Loss, pain, insecurity maybe even despair begins to engulf you. Your mentors urge you to carry on with life as you struggle for survival. You believe it is the worst possible thing that ever happened to you until—the penetrating piercing ring of the phone awakens you from a deep sleep in the middle of the night. You instantly know this cannot be encouraging as your heart races and you struggle to reach the receiver. On the other end of the line, you hear your daughter hysterically informing you that your son-in-law has shot himself and is on the way to the emergency room. Your mind blindly races for the right response. You attempt to calm her while trying to compose yourself by reaching out to the only strength in your life you've ever trusted, Jesus. You pray.

You tell her you're on your way. You pray. You frantically get dressed, you pray. You rush to your car into the silent dark of the night while the rest of the world is peacefully slumbering. You pray. Traveling a non-congested highway the car and your thoughts racing you pray. What else would you do? "God, please let him live!" Oh God, if he is hurt bad, if he is going to be a vegetable, take him—Oh

God, no this can't be happening. Please guide my daughter, oh my God my grandson, Oh God?" You just pray.

I still feel the pain today, as I write. I had previously thought the darkest time of my life was experiencing divorce and the loss of custody of my children. Nothing, absolutely nothing to this point was more devastating than watching my child, now grown, experience the suicide of my grandson's father. Those moments long past are not just a blur in my memory, they are vivid and painful. Arriving at the emergency entrance, the scene I witnessed was unbelievable. The vast number of friends and family gathered there sobbing and consoling one another was overwhelmingly phenomenal. Instinctively, I knew at that moment he didn't make it. I again, prayed. However, the worst moments were yet to be endured, the identification of his body and ultimately then heading back to my daughter's home to awaken my grandson and tell him his father was gone. He was only a child, a young unsuspecting child who loved his Dad. I continuously prayed for his family, my family and all those who were grieving. I comforted, cried and loved by God's grace as much as I could. At this writing it has been over two and one half years now and every time my grandson reaches a new milestone in his life without his father present, I still grieve and I still pray.

In those deep, dark and devastating moments, what riches you might ask? What if there had been nowhere to turn, no one to pray to, no grace, no strength, no guidance? My daughter today, has stronger Faith, turning to the rock in times of trouble. Taking her anger, disappointment and fear and laying them at the foot of the cross, as she has been taught. She prays, an answer to a mother's lifetime of prayer. She and others through that terrible experience found comfort in each other and in God.

She has ministered strength and Faith to her son, to his mother and sister in their time of grief. My pastor ministered hope to over three hundred grieving friends, family and co-workers. A family deep in despair were brought closer to each other by God and to God. Many riches were discovered in the deepest depths of darkness, so all would know that He is Lord. He makes streams out of wastelands, and rivers of life out of dry ground. He came to set the captives free and heal the broken hearted. If it had not been for the

Lord on our side the raging torrents of deep despair would certainly have swept us away. We discovered family is a treasure to behold that may slip too easily from our fingers and we hold on tighter.

Just recently I had the privilege to view a video that was emailed by my daughter[bless this modern technology]. I had been unable to make it to my grandson's track meet so she taped it with her camera. The video allowed me to experience something I never would have had the opportunity to do in person from the bleachers at the track meet. View my grandson *close up* as he ran the Sprint. Way out in front, he set a record that day as he won that race. What I saw however, was the emotion in his face, the determination in his Spirit up close and personal! I saw his dad, a runner also in his high school days. I saw a young boy determined to win a race for his father and I know he will be just as determined to win the race of life, and finish his course. I pray.

In loving memory of Michael J. Mosher Jr., January 31, 1976 to April 9, 2005.

Chapter Two

Adjust Your Spiritual Eyes

Look to the Light to illuminate the pathway. God will give us a glimmer of light; sometimes it takes a moment in time for our spiritual eyes to adjust. Today, is Father's Day, I am reminded this morning that Faith does not believe in a God that can, it believes in a God that will!

Pastor James E. Holder has been my spiritual father, pastor, mentor, teacher and beloved friend for almost thirteen years of my spiritual walk. Through many fires I have escaped unscathed because of his faithfulness to preach the Gospel of Christ unabridged. Currently, I face another sea to cross, adversities to overcome. Do I believe God can? Absolutely, I have been taught well and the last several chapters have certainly shown evidence of the times He did. Believing that God can and believing that God will are a smidgen different. The "will" in that statement depends upon our ability to believe we are worthy to receive that blessing. Believing that one more time, he will again see us through. One more time His patience will prevail. One more time He will release His mercy and grace. One more time His assistance to clean up the mess we have created will be present. Are you willing to receive?

How do we convince our doubting minds that He will? Simple, it is written in scripture.

Matthew 7:7 versus 9-11 "Ask, and it shall be given you; seek, and ye shall find; knock, and it shall be opened unto you, Or what man is there of you, whom if his son ask bread, will he give him a stone? Or if he ask a fish, will he give him a serpent? If ye then, being evil, know how to give good gifts unto your children, how much more shall your Father which is in heaven give good things to them that ask him?" KJV

2 Corinthians 12:9 "and he said unto me, My grace is sufficient for thee: for my strength is made perfect in weakness." KJV

The word says it and I believe it. Do you? In our weakest moments as we appeal to the faithfulness of God and His word, He makes His grace available to us just for the asking. We accomplish many things we never dreamed we would. Those who trust in Him cannot be shaken no matter what the force. If you are still having difficulty, I empathize. There are times when we are flooded in darkness and focusing becomes complex. We may suffer from Spiritual Astigmatism. Our spiritual eyes may need adjustment. In the natural, as we walk into a very dark room coming from the light, it takes time for our eyes to adjust to darkness. Initially, it is difficult to see anything, but gradually our eyes will adjust and things surrounding us become clearer to our vision.

God will give you a glimmer of light in the darkness, illuminate your path and lead you through even the toughest of times. Earlier, I shared briefly the parental circumstance of my childhood. My biological father abandoning me as a toddler leaving a scar of insecurity and worthlessness and a belief that were I of any value or significance he would have stayed to love and care for me. My step-father, an alcoholic and emotionally distant at times added to that belief. So initially, Father's Day was a difficult time. Thank God for the unhidden riches, my grandfather who filled the gap. I constantly struggled with the concept of Fatherhood and perception of a loving protective Father. With an also emotionally distant mother, I craved love, attention and acceptance. I gave my grandfather the love and respect due him each year as Father's Day rolled around but I ignored how cheated I felt and resigned myself to the situation. I quickly developed the "poor me" syndrome and became self-serving and independent. I didn't at the time see the hidden riches in a loving God-fearing grandfather provided by God himself to offer me what I needed. It was also hard to see God as loving and protecting at that time.

Introduced to church at a young age, I clung to the words of that old hymn: "Yes, Jesus loves me, the Bible tells me so". At last, someone loves even me. Later going to a Catholic church with my friends my religious education changed direction. The concept of The Heavenly Father became one of strict discipline and penance. I was in awe but afraid of failing, afraid of sinning and afraid of abandonment by God also. I began to search several religions and finally found what I was looking for. Yes, He is a Holy God, a loving God. Yes, He expects adherence to His commands and yes He disciplines us in love. Has He ever abandoned me? Never and I am aware that His word says He never will. My Father loves me now, just as I am but too much to leave me the way I am. He gave me a grandfather to guide the way through life. I give Him my life, he disciplines because He loves me and allows adversity to strengthen me, trials to teach me, loss that I might gain and loneliness that I might seek Him.

John 10:17-18 "The Father loves me because I lay down my life that I may have it back again." TLB

1 John 4:10 "This is love: not that we loved God, but that he loved us and sent his Son as an atoning sacrifice for our sins." NIV

Happy Father's Day Abba Father! June 17, 2007

Hold To God's Unchanging Hand. In this life the only constant is change. In Michigan, the Water Wonderland where I reside things are always changing. In relationship to driving we have two seasons: Winter and Construction. You are either faced with the challenge of maneuvering around snow, ice and slush or those awful orange cones in construction zones. If you don't like the weather you only need to wait a day or two and it will change. The thermometer may register 80 degrees one day and 40 the next, literally! We have had snow in June and tornadoes in December.

I love the seasonal changes, but we have changes within the changes. All summer long, traffic routes will constantly change due to construction. One day you find a route around it thinking you have hit the jackpot and the next the dreaded orange barrels appear meaning road repairs ahead expect detours. Life for some of us is much the same, ever-changing. One week things are stable you find a way to survive, the next turmoil.

As I complete this chapter I am awaiting, believing and expecting miracles. Remember those divine interventions by the hand of God that makes a change in our circumstance? Notice that miracle is plural, I believe I need more than one. Why? Recently, I was terminated from a professional position for providing information to authorities regarding legal violations. My only income and on the same day I took ill, which was later diagnosed as kidney stones and an ovarian tumor. At my age there should not be an ovary left to have a tumor. But, Tell that to the ovary.

I have since experienced several months with no income along with the adversity at hand. Gaining assistance from state agencies proved to be futile for one reason or another. It did not take long to deplete what little savings I had, ruin my credit standing and become delinquent with bills. Down to my last dollar and facing eviction I knew God could change the circumstance. I did all the right things, I prayed, sought His help, listened, read the word, cried and nothing changed. In some circumstances things worsened. I asked others to pray, they did, little changed. I verbalized Faith: "God will make a way, His promises are true and I believe in Miracles." Truly, I believed He could, today I know I may have been questioning if He would. Today, I know He will, in His way, in His time! Where does our help come from, anyway?

Psalm 121:1-2 "I lift my eyes to the hills, where does my help come from? My help comes from the LORD, the Maker of heaven and earth." NIV

Pastor seemed confident the whole time and gave me four words: "It's a fixed fight". I ended up with *two* law firms to represent me, received checks from friends and unknowns, found a teaching position I love to this day and registered my first business. Not too mention, plenty of free time to write and minister, the passion of my life. He turned around what the enemy meant for evil into something wonderful.

God is faithful, a miracle did occur which due to legal grounds I am not at liberty to share the outcome. Trust me, He does the impossible. The Word confirms it somewhat like this. Those who trust in the Lord are like Mount Zion they cannot be shaken! As the old hymn says and my pastor often sings: "Hold to God's Unchanging Hand".

Chapter Three

Slow Down, Detour Ahead

A s I completed the last chapter with renewed hope and faith believing I did not know that things were about to become a bit more challenging. Did I just describe the challenge as a "bit"? How unusual for a writer to minimize a situation rather than embellish it. It has become considerably more challenging to say the least. Too much for me in fact, but thankfully not too much for my God. There are three major defeating attitudes or obstacles to reaching our destiny that we have previously touched upon. If we are not careful they dash our expectations, crowd out our hope and threaten to diminish our Faith. For summarization purposes let me repeat them. Fear, Discouragement, and Offense. It almost overtook me this past week. Hopefully, you will by my experience be able to avoid the same type of diversion.

It was a hot, humid, typical Michigan-July morning. As I awoke I could see the steamy hot weather from inside my air-conditioned window. Thank you Lord, for air-conditioning and how blessed I was that my electricity was still on to run it. I hastily said a few prayers, my first mistake. Never let your prayer time be hasty. Jumped out of bed with anticipation for today was the day I would finally put into action the plans I had carefully laid for my new business. The manual was complete. Fifteen employees of the facility I was servicing would be called in for the In-Service I would teach. Excited and a bit anxious, I ignored the nagging colicky pain in my right lower quadrant of my abdomen, my second mistake. By the time I picked up Ashleigh, my videographer for the day and headed to the facility I had made several stops to a restroom as the pain was increasing in intensity. I arrived on time however, gritting my teeth and clenching the chair next to me I began the presentation with less than normal enthusiasm. After excusing myself more than once to utilize their restroom facilities it became increasingly apparent that I would need to postpone the next two hours of teaching to be on my way to the nearest emergency facility. I did just that worrying and fretting over the future of my new business. I never did confront a detour with style. I was impatient and irritated.

Awaiting results after examinations, x-rays and cat scans; I was not sure which was more grave. The reason for the excruciating pain or the fact that with no insurance I would have to pay the resulting bill. A diagnosis of Kidney Stones, and Ovarian Cyst definitely was not something to shout about or maybe it was. Since that time, one stone has passed but the large one had lodged itself in such a position that required visits to a specialist who recommended a surgical procedure to place a stent to allow the stone opening to pass through. To some that may not sound so disheartening, but with no insurance, to me it was. I found myself fighting even more intensely with those revolting obstacles that I now try to avoid, discouragement and fear!

As if that were not enough, the adversary found ways to throw in criticism from friends and offense for good measure. I turned the situation over to God though the battle was not an easy one. Already facing court dates, loss of my home and credit rating; now my health also was threatening to overwhelm me. I took a stand and please note I would not recommend such drastic measures to everyone. You must be in a place where you know that you know that you know, God is leading you to extend your Faith. I made the decision to completely place my healing into the hands of the almighty physician. If my God who can do all things cannot remove this stone from where it is lodged than neither can a surgical procedure which is risky and will assure my financial demise. I refused surgery and placed the situation into the hands of God. Scripture assures me that God can do all things according to His riches in Glory and in this case the riches were mine to claim and that I did. He did exceedingly abundantly more than I asked. I determined that unless He told me differently, I would trust Him to do spiritual radical surgery not only on my body but my heart. He did it for others why not me? I believed He would{He eventually did}.

I did not get to this place in my walk of Faith without struggle, mentoring, prayer or without determination. It was difficult to fathom that this was happening just when I thought I was almost there{By the way we are never there}. It was detour on the journey to my destiny that served to remind me that this road to God's planned purpose for our lives is just that. A journey not a destination. Yes, I was annoyed at first, in fact, I did not realize how angry. I was dismayed for sure, I definitely did not desire to face another detour. That anger surfaced one Sunday morning unexpectedly. I begrudgingly awoke from a fretful nights' sleep. My precious, friend and companion, Gus was pestering me to let him outside to relieve himself. He was not pleased with my hesitant and leisurely arousal and chose to relieve himself on my briefcase. Not only did the deafening and piercing "No!" surprise me but sent him dashing tail between his legs to hide from the witch from whence it came. This was the ultimate insult, all that I was enduring and now was being peed upon by my best friend.

You may be laughing right now, I was not. I was humiliated and angry. Had this not all begun with my representing integrity, doing the right thing. I was losing everything and self-pity over road me as I played back the whole past four months. Hospital visits, hours of working through pages and pages of interrogatories detailing my life since high school. Do you know how long ago that was? Constant calls from creditors. I had believed God for miracles, where were they?

The end result of all this surfacing turmoil was a cup heaved with vengeance into the sink smashing into splintered fragments about the kitchen. I burst into tears and faced the fact that this non-violent, faith-filled Christian woman was angry! Gus had enough dog-sense to stay in a place of safety and eventually so did I. I cried my heart out, quickly dressed in what was the closest thing I could find and with no make up ran to my place of safety. Church{Pity those who had to look at me}.

Yes, it was a detour on the road to purpose, but ever so necessary for me to recognize a weakness. I had found a way to conquer fear, knowing that power, love and a sound mind was mine to claim and walk in. I had hung on with all my strength and God's to hope and overcame discouragement. I thought I had let go of offense, forgiven and moved on. Apparently not! It had only taken an indiscretion by my little friend Gus to expose what lay beneath and bring my anger to the surface. I was still hurting at the injustice of the deeds of the offenders. I was outraged at the audacity of their request to question my life and integrity. In case you are wondering, Yes, Gus has forgiven me. I guess that is why they call dogs man's best friend.

Philippians 3:13 "Brethren, I do not consider myself as having attained but[this]one thing[I do] forgetting those things that are behind, and reaching forth to those things that are ahead, I press toward the mark for the prize of the high calling of God in Christ Jesus."

It is indeed frustrating when you are on a journey so close to your destination or at least what you believe is your destination, only to come across a detour that takes you off the main road. You have planned, anticipated and envisioned how and how long it will take you to reach your desired destination. Suddenly, a detour guides you in a new direction and you proceed in unfamiliar territory, unsure of your direction, delayed and possibly dismayed. There may or may not be others traveling with you also irritated at the unexpected turn of events making their frustrations well known. Suddenly, powerlessness overtakes you as you realize you no longer have control of the journey. Is not that the very reason for your frustration, you are no longer in control.

Powerlessness is not always a negative connotation, it simply means a power greater is in control. If we allow it that power can be God. In reality, detours have a common purpose. Possibly a bridge is out and to continue on the chosen path could prove disastrous. Maybe the current road is full of potholes, unsafe and in need of repair so to continue your journey could cause further delay or harm. Or perhaps a new road is in the process of construction which when finished will provide safer travel for future journeys. We often do not consider the future journeys because our focus is limited to the here and now. Instant gratification, we want to get where we are going and get there immediately if not sooner! In our spiritual walk detours represent similar issues, our chosen path may bring about future disaster, or the road so full of unsafe and hazardous circumstances that to continue would do great harm. Possibly God has a new direction providing blessing along the way or at a future time. We would do best to consider a detour a blessing in disguise.

I once read an awesome piece on Detours written by Les Crause. He made a great point as he wrote that we often set goals and make plans from the vision God has given, further he states that if you have committed those plans to the Lord and asked in Faith and accordance to the Word, you can be sure He has set in motion plans to cause these things to come about. Thank you Les for opening my eyes and teaching me to recognize when the plans *you* {the key here is the you} had suddenly change or you hit a detour, what will your attitude be? He also pointed out that reflection upon the detour is necessary. It is necessary and if reflected upon immediately and with openness his purpose will be revealed. Ask yourself, is it of the Lord, the world, or the enemy?

Chapter Four

October's Child

In order to describe the *riches* I discovered *stored in secret places* and conclude the writing of this book, I need to back-track a few years. It lead me on a fifteen-year journey that taught me the lessons learned that I have openly shared in the past chapters with you. My own roller coaster ride through relationships of domestic violence, family alcoholism, abandonment and divorce.

In October of 1995, as the leaves in Michigan attained the peak of their brilliant color, the course of my life suddenly took a razor-sharp turn. I took a short sabbatical from my position as a Detox Supervisor to participate in a revival week-end as a part of a two-hundred person choir. It was Sweetest Day week-end as well. As the conference was coming to a close, a call was made by the Revival Evangelist to the choir members to submit a long-desired prayer request. He assured us as we wrote our requests that finding favor with our service to Him, God was going to move in these situations according to His perfect will. He encouraged us to submit our request in Faith believing that what we asked for would indeed come to pass. I had been living the lonely life of a single woman far too long and in Faith and desperation I prayed for a husband! *Warning:* Be careful what you pray for, you may just obtain it!

I drove home at the commencement of the conference with a friend who had attended with me. Metaphorically speaking, I was flying at least a foot off the ground though in reality one of them was heavy on the pedal. Thus my nickname that week-end became "Andretti". It had been a wonderful week-end and I was on a spiritual high like I had never experienced. Unfortunately, all things that go up must come down. I believe they call it gravity. Well, the gravity of the situation was that I was now home, alone, and on Sweetest Day.

I was extremely aware that I was no longer in such an awesome presence of God. It was amazing how deeply I felt that loss. As that awareness began to overwhelm me, the loss of God's presence and my selfish desire to share a day of love with someone, it translated itself into profound sobbing. The overwhelming sense of emptiness turned into self-pity and an increased desire for someone to comfort me. A husband. After all, is that not what woman was created for? Little did I know the fulfillment of my desire and prayer [my future mate] was soon to present itself.

On Monday following however, the manifestation of that dream walked into my life. He was not exactly what I had envisioned. For years I had a list of all the qualities I desired in a mate. A list so ideal that only Jesus Christ himself could possibly have fulfilled it. What can I say? My past experiences were so disappointing that I was aiming high!

He was not at all what I expected. Oh, He was handsome and humorous. But, He was an alcoholic who had decided to enter into our treatment center to become sober the very day I had attended the conference. Saturday, October 21, 1995, not only was that Sweetest Day, it was also his birthday that year! So he had decided to begin life anew.

I did not come face-to-face with him until later that Monday. Still floating from my wonderful week-end experience I breezed through the usual daily tasks of the treatment center. The only difference I was smiling, happy and focused on Spiritual things. Toward the end of the workday, I was approached by a fellow employee. He requested that I speak to a gentlemen who was leaving treatment without an after-care plan {my responsibility} prior to his scheduled out-date. I agreed and we came *face to face*. He was at the time, not someone I would have taken a second look at. Heavy-bearded with silvery grey hair, he could have passed for Father Time.

His face was rugged and as russet as the turning leaves outside the window. His articulate conversation brisk as the October winds. His demeanor as determined and certain as the onset of Winter that currently was threatening our doorstep. As sure as he was born within the month, he was definitely October's child.

My usual success at convincing a client not to leave treatment early was to no avail with this determined man. He had a plan and a story and he was sticking to it! I became aware of his compassionate nature though as he shared the urgent need to return to four dependent cats awaiting his arrival home. He had rescued everyone of them as abandoned kittens and now was concerned for their welfare. As I write that, need I mention I think he had me hooked from that moment though I didn't realize it at the time. Discharge planning led to a dialogue of a divine nature which often occurred due to the spirituality of the 12-step program.

It was also disclosed that I had previously met him three years earlier when he came to pick up his brother after a stay in our program. His recollection stirred my memory of that time and his brother. He shared the respect and admiration he had felt for me at that time, while also commenting positively with regard to my current countenance. I believe he used the word, "glowing". He was impressed by my Faith and inquired as to my beliefs and the religious institution I attended. I explained that I was a part of a non-denominational church and believed not in a religion but in a personal relationship with Christ. He then asked for the address of the church and was informed that I could not refer him specifically to "my church" due to company regulation, but could offer him a list of churches mine included from which he could make a personal choice. He acknowledged his understanding of our protocol, took the referrals and left to attend to his home, his sobriety and his beloved cats. I received beautifully written letters from him that week alluding to our conversations.

The following Wednesday evening I attended our usual church services. A delightful and spirited elderly gentlemen, David Sharpe was filling in that night with an evangelistic message concerning the willingness of Christ to accept us just as we are. A moving message to say the least that consequently drew several persons to the altar.

I had been sitting up front in the first pew to avoid distractions as I usually do. I was totally unaware of who might be seated behind me in the church. As the altar call progressed, I noticed the elderly gentlemen trying to get up from the altar on his own and proceeded forward to give him assistance. I was helping him to his feet as an obvious incident was occurring nearby. I could overhear the Pastor tell the congregation that the young man in front of him had just rededicated his life to the Lord and renounced his bondage to alcoholism. Hearing the word alcoholism, I turned quickly in that direction. As the man turned toward me I gazed into the most piercing sapphire-blue eyes you have ever seen enhanced only by the silvery grey hair above them! They had the clarity and luster of Lake Tahoe on the clearest of days. A lightening bolt went straight to my heart and left its mark forever.

It was him. I did not recognize him at first, though he had silvery grey hair. This night, it was neatly cut and groomed and his face clean-shaven. His smile sent a radiance across the room that engulfed my entire being and left an afterglow. I had not felt this way in years, was it the Spirit, was it me or was it love at first sight? It later became apparent after speaking with him, that this was October's child, the man from treatment earlier that week. I was immediately drawn to him and the red flags surfaced immediately! A recovering alcoholic, single for many years, independent and determined, watch out. I was a counselor, I knew better. My heart won out and I didn't listen to wisdom. After a whirlwind courtship chaperoned the whole time, we were married the following May, 1996 seven months later. He remained true to my description, strong-minded, confident and in control; but warm, compassionate and loving at times.

With the good qualities unfortunately he carried deep devastating wounds of the past that served to rear their ugly head from time to time. We had three good years together and then the predictable came to pass. The alcoholic personality and stinkin-thinkin surfaced. He respected me enough to protect me and leave our homestead as he became angry, out-of-control, and abusive. He knew those were the times when in order to break away from the overwhelming emotions of daily living he would eventually escape into a swirling-devouring bottle of alcohol. His control would lapse into months of non-control.

When he would return I would willingly welcome him with open arms and extend my love and forgiveness. I know I did this out of a past deep-desire to see loved ones overcome the world of addiction and find true freedom in the savior I knew so well. I really believed against all that I was taught, that if I just showed him the love of Christ in me it would change him. However, this proved to be the pattern every few years of our life until my patience and his ran out. He gave up, I gave in. We decided to separate our physical-living by a divorce. We remained best-friends always and the love for him never left my heart.

I buried my love for him profoundly deep within or so I thought, by serving others at work, in the ministry and keeping extremely busy. We saw each other frequently as friends only and he stayed away during an alcoholic drinking binge for two to three months at a time.

October's child evolved into a period of profound sullenness and emptiness much like the Michigan Winter does after a Fall Harvest. In the Spring he would always find new life again. New hope would bud forth and bring fruit until the following Fall. A journey repeated many times over in our moments-in-time together. I never stopped seeking God for a miracle in his life, however I did give-up on believing for restoration of our marriage. I continued on my journey to discover my destiny and my desire to have a loving god-fearing husband some day. I opened my mouth many a time speaking it forth and looking for it to come to pass. Especially in the Spring when the long dreary Winter has passed and hope of new life literally springs forth.

Psalm 81:10 "I am the Lord thy God who brought thee up out of the land of Egypt: Open thy mouth wide and I will fill it"

What an encouragement to pray! We ask such undersized things because our thinking is so small but the LORD would have us request great blessings. Prayer should be as simple a matter as the opening of the mouth. It should be a natural unconstrained utterance.

Speaking of having desire and opening of mouths. Have you ever noticed a nest of new baby birds in the spring? Neither their wings nor their judgment is developed enough to fly or search for food. As the mother bird approaches the nest with a worm in her mouth, instantaneously their mouths gape wide open with expectancy. She drops the worm into their anxiously awaiting beaks and no sooner has the chosen one swallowed his dinner than his mouth begins to gape open once more! Off again and again she flies to satisfy their insatiable hunger.

We would all do well to approach the possession of our desires, the possession of our inheritance with the same expectancy and enthusiasm. We need to enlarge the scope of our thinking, while reaching out to gain new perspectives and great victories! There are large victories to be won, enlarge the scope of your vision. We lose perspective and instead of stepping forward into our next place of victory we lose our footing. Open your mouth wide with expectation and receive. So I did continuously call unto God to change him.

Jeremiah 33:3 "Call to me and I will answer you and tell you great and unsearchable things you do not know"

Things you do not know, riches hidden in secret places. Declare to the Heavens your destiny awaits, your miracle is complete. Why then was I believing for my husband's deliverance and not believing for marriage restoration? I have learned that most of the time the obstacles that appear in my life come from my previous life decisions. I know the Lord sees the whole picture whether there be a detour or traffic jam, or a boulder blocking our path, another mountain to climb. He knows what is ahead, I only see what is directly in front of me, I understand now that the detours, the delays along the journey to fulfillment are meant to strengthen not to harm me. I also realize that sometimes the obstacle is not always about me and that always all things are for the Glory of God to be shown in the circumstance. Eventually, it will come to an end. Yes, dear friend Sally, "This too shall pass!"

There are innumerable times in each life when without our choice we are faced with the necessity of letting go, beginning anew. Endings actually are beginnings backwards if you think about it. As you move on to open a new door you must close the old one. Leaving things behind is heartrending however unlocking new horizons in the future fulfilling. As I come to the end of our journey together and the end of this book, I have let go. However, I am awaiting a miraculous supernatural intervention of God.

It is not an end but a beginning of a new chapter in life. I still have a need, I still have desires and God is able to supply them. I believe He will! I will not focus on the massive stones blocking the passageway. I carry within my backpack, energy and Faith to remove the hindrances I may discover in the climb upward. In my powerlessness to control or change the circumstances my cries have not gone unheard. Our loving savior has an advanced plan and step-by-step as I seek guidance, it will unfold. The obstacles with His help will be removed. The detour will come to an end and I will be on a familiar road again. The boulder piece by piece will be chipped away until I can walk over or around it or with the help of others push it aside. The broken areas I thought I could not cross over only to find just around the bend a bridge that as I take each step is built under my feet.

He will transform your valley of troubles into a path of hope, free you from captivity. Though the process has been long, or difficult I am reminded that with each step I am nearer the threshold. I am reminded that though I no longer have that physical bridegroom to carry me over it is time to let the Lord do so. He has promised to show me *Riches Stored in Secret Places*. He has. *Treasures of Darkness*, He has. He will because I believe He will! He is God and this is just....

The Beginning.

Epilogue

The Rest of The Story

Nine months ago I completed Treasures and prepared to send it for publication, but forces kept me from doing so. With immense passion I can say that from conception it was a labor of love that produced many months of anticipation, growth and new life. Delivery was imminent and enduring Faith has ensued. In the past year of tolerated affliction, I discovered the most delightful reassurance. Hopefully, it will also be of some comfort as you face trials that shake you to core; the kind that rattles your brain, distorts your visions and leaves answers unclear. When your efforts are exhausted and you are no longer holding on by a thread remember He is holding you.

Some of you have been tested and tried far greater than others. The great British Baptist Preacher, Charles Spurgeon once said: "Some are tried very specially that is because God has a great favour to them." It is just evidence of His great love for you, a love that surpasses all others!

Revelation 3:19 "As many as I love, I rebuke and chasten"

Are We There Yet?

Don't you just love it when your child keeps asking on a journey, Dad are we there yet? I am sure our Heavenly Father God feels exactly the same when we think we have things all figured out and

He has additional plans for us. I thought I was finished and had concluded the last chapter of this book. Well, God had further plans. Just when you think you are finished you are not finished. So here goes, a destiny revealed.

When I started writing this book 3 years ago, I had every intention of completing it within a year; I had no idea at the time that I would be living it while I was writing it. Thinking that the experiential lessons I desired to share were already learned I was anxious to move it to completion. I now know why it was unfinished, there was yet another treasure still buried.

I have shared many life experiences along with their subsequent lessons to this point. However, the one I am about to share is the most excruciating yet most rewarding of all, unfortunately also very recent.

In April of 2008, I finally received a call from my estranged husband, Michael. It had been the longest period of silence yet about 5 months. It appeared a miracle had taken place and he shared an awesome personal experience he had had with the Lord. His intention, he told me, was to return to our church that night and begin again living his life in the footsteps of Christ. He did just that!

The following Saturday, a beautiful breezy afternoon I traveled with Michael to a place well visited by us on the St. Clair River. The river showed the brilliance of a dazzling sapphire as it reflected the blue of the sky overhead. Sitting on a bench on the boardwalk we watched the cargo ships pass by and talked for hours. Something in him had changed it was obvious, but would it be enough to sustain him in his desired Christian-walk this time? I was more than slightly skeptical. His demeanor was still controlled but with animation. As we left the pier, we made plans to meet at church the next morning and have lunch following services. I had no idea what was in store for me and therefore was caught completely off guard.

Sunday after a wonderful service, lunch and light-hearted spiritual conversation he dropped me off at home asking permission to come in and use the restroom facilities. Afterward, following a hug [not unusual] as he left my doorstep to proceed to his vehicle something in the atmosphere surrounding us changed drastically. It truly was as if The Spirit's arrow [not cupid's] of undeniable love had been shot simultaneously into both our hearts at the same moment. I turned on the steps, he moved toward me. I moved down the steps as if controlled by something other than myself and he moved closer coming toward me. Suddenly, cupping my chin in his hand he bent down and kissed me ever so slightly on the chin[not usual]. Those striking blue eyes dazzling and an mischievous grin, he walked to his truck.

I floated six inches off the ground I am sure into the house thinking: Oh no! God this cannot be happening again. I cannot walk this path again. No sooner did the thoughts enter my mind than the shrill of the cell phone brought me back to reality. Michael's voice was filled with confidence and speculation as he said, "I know you and I know what you're thinking, you're pacing up and down telling God you can't do this again and questioning how this can be happening. Stop worrying Terry, just let go and let God."

He was right. I was pacing and worrying. I was not ready to open my heart to him just to be crushed again. I had not realized the love I still harbored until it came flooding from the depths of my heart with the force of a giant Tsunami. Yet, I knew the power drawing us together was much stronger than we were and my heart told me this was of God even though it made little logical sense. To many others in the weeks that followed it didn't either and they did not hesitate to make their concerns well known.

The days, weeks and months that followed were unsurpassed by any that I had experienced in years prior and I will cherish the memories of them in the years to come. It was a spiritual high. A time overflowing with joy, laughter, love and peace. They were wonderful times walking, sharing spiritual insights, watching the birds, and the roll of the waves at Metropolitan Beach. Exploring the property where he grew up in Romeo and sharing pleasant memories of his childhood. Planning a future including those things we had missed out on. A fulfillment of all my hopes, dreams and prayers. A restorative miracle. We were remarried in August and moved to a beautiful rural home together along with four cats and one dog and we lived happily ever after. If this were a fairy tale maybe, but...

Initially, we were unable to move in together with two separate living spaces to dispose of. When that was taken care of we packed up and set upon a new chapter of our journey. The first day of moving in together the enemy came in like flood and that could fill another book. Just like Murphy's Law, What could go wrong did and the battle raged on. Darkness settled over us to depths that to this day are beyond description. Michael began to struggle with the enemy not only for sobriety but for his very life, eternal life. The attack upon him was relentless and at times it appeared he was losing the battle. I struggled to function, hold onto my faith and minister to him. A prophecy had been given to us with regard to serving in a ministerial capacity to those in bondage to addiction and as we set it in motion the battle became even more fierce!

Exhausted I sunk into a deep-depression like I had never experienced. I had had everything I dreamed of in my fingertips and now it was slipping away. I was overwhelmed by the fear that once again I would lose him and everything else. Not to mention that other areas of my life proved challenging concurrently. Would he overcome, would I? For the first time in a very long time in my spiritual journey I was doubting. Consequently I felt I had no one to turn to. My family had been skeptical in the first place, I didn't feel I could even tell them. Our decision to reunite and our faith that God would restore our relationship had been questioned by most of our friends, they wouldn't understand. My closest friend at the time was overwhelmed with issues of her own and beside herself as to how to help me. She couldn't and didn't. There was one exception, our pastor. Even so, he was concerned with regard to the seriousness of my depression and recommended counseling. I was horrified and refused. After all I was a counselor and a minister I did not need counseling. I was just discouraged and so I sunk lower. I can honestly say it was the second time in my life I really no longer wanted to live.

I truly do not remember the defining moment that snapped me back to reality, enough to fight back. Maybe, it was just the simple cry for help and God's faithful response. Be that as it may, it changed my life completely and forevermore. Actually, it is one of the most remarkable life-changing times yet. The Lord used several methods to demonstrate to me that the one thing my husband needed from me most was unconditional love. True Agape Love not my feeble attempts that I call sloppy agape. You know the kind I mean. "Oh yes dear, I love you. I love you unconditionally" We do until they do something that we disagree with or become angry with. Unconditional means just that unconditional! No demands, no ifs, no buts, love no matter what. No conditions attached. He set me out on a mission to learn and apply.

The significant change came about one morning extremely early. After all isn't that the time God usually chooses to speak to us, very early? Through scripture, study and prayer I knew that I was going to truly have to sacrifice my desires [not needs, He supplies all our needs] to minister to those of my husbands'. I loved him enough but was I unselfish enough? The Lord inspired me to begin a challenge to our church members to grow in tolerance for others by putting together a 40 day love-challenge fast during Lent. Not the push aside the TV or meal kind. Not a giving up but a determining to do, kind. Through the help of scriptures a fast to determine to perform daily random acts of kindness and/or forgiveness. He motivated me one week at a time which I presented to the congregation each Sunday morning. Many others joined with me in this challenge and the results were welcome responses by the recipients of our acts of kindness.

During about the third week of the Love challenge, my husband and I made a trip to the local Christian book store and I came across a video, which we purchased, took home and viewed together. "Fireproof". What an awesome discovery and challenge to our marriage and confirmation that I was indeed hearing from God. It was obvious at the time that I was slightly more impressed by the movie than Michael but never-the-less I knew I would purchase the journal mentioned in the movie anyway.

The next week I did purchase "The Love Dare" journal written by Stephen and Alex Kendrick with Lawrence Kimbrough. One of the first dares to be presented in the book was to say nothing negative to your spouse and do at least one unexpected gesture as an act of kindness. I didn't find it too difficult in the beginning to follow the suggestions and journal the feelings and results. However, as time went on the challenges became more difficult for me. I was not seeing results or at least so I thought at the time. It is hard to demonstrate love to others when you are not encouraged to do so. But I was determined and I learned so much from the process. I learned that Agape Love was far more than unconditional, it actually was a God-love and it would take God to help me bestow it upon Michael. I was forced to keep conscious-contact with the Lord at all times to maintain my quest. In the meantime, I was still completing the challenge with the church.

My greatest goal in my Christian walk is to become a Proverbs 31 woman. It was always to be godly wife and mother. I desired a loving husband, a solid marriage and godly home to minister love and direction to my children and grandchildren. I wanted peace, no conflict and joy. Now, who doesn't? I was willing to sacrifice anything to experience at least a portion of my dream and remember I do believe in miracles. So I committed to the Lord to maintain this forty-day Love Dare, determined to see it through no matter what. I truly believed my next miracle was on its way and if I were just obedient, the demons plaguing us would let go and my marriage vision would resume.

Those of you who have lived in the hellish grips of addiction know the movement through the honeymoon, eggshell, relapse stages. My spirit knew with dread and trepidation that relapse was imminent and it was not long before my loving husband was transformed into a dark controlling stranger who made the decision to move out while still assuring me of his love. He justified his current abandonment with explanations of his need to keep his life simple to avoid relapse and the overwhelming challenges and difficulties that had plagued us since moving into a home. He assured me our relationship would be better than ever before and divorce was not an option. Two days after moving he relapsed and began a 3 week binge drowning himself in alcohol daily like so many times before.

The difference this time was that I was prepared to find the Treasure of Darkness and willing to search in hidden places for riches. The difference this time, me. I was saddened yes! Determined definitely, I was not angry. My friends and family were. I was not willing to give up on him. Almost everyone else was. Disappointed along with them, I also knew his health would not tolerate too many more assaults against it. I cried, I moved out of the nightmare house and I kept constant contact. Eventually, he became sick enough [I like to use the phrase so far down there is no where else to look but up] to ask for help, from me, God and finally our pastor.

He sobered up, returned to church and began his journey again. He shared testimony that while seeking Christ's forgiveness he clearly heard the choice given to him. Do you want to live or die? He clearly heard the Lord tell him that this would be the **last time**, he was not to drink again. He shared these intimate realizations openly and stated at one point: "Life is Life, Life changes. Drunks are Drunks because they won't accept reality so they try to create their own controlled world". I believe it and truly what he had lived by to this point. All was well for awhile and he was right. Our relationship was better than ever. His beloved father passed on to eternity in December and my concern heightened as to his ability to handle such a devastating loss. His health was deteriorating and the added stress was of no help. I sensed a change in his resolve as he took measures consecutively to arrange dinners with his closest friends on Tuesday and Wednesday on my birthday with me.

Then on Friday, January 29, 2010, a few months ago my high hopes took a sudden nosedive. I received a call from my daughter that her beloved pregnant friend since junior high was dying of a brain aneurysm. She and the infant did not survive. Michael called to inform me that he had picked up drinking alcohol once again and we both knew it would be his last drunk.

I spent the next two weeks checking on him daily and watching him quickly deteriorate. At the end of the week, I felt a strong urging in my spirit to make plans to stay with him at his apartment for the week-end as he kept telling me he was not going to make it this time. He felt he did not have long to live. He wanted to reach a sober state first. If he was able, he also wanted to accomplish some things with me that were desires of mine. He stopped drinking on Thursday evening. On Friday morning, I packed an overnight bag and headed to his apartment. I had been making daily cell phone contact with my mentor and friend as I traveled to see him expecting to find him lifeless and this morning was no different. I called Sally that morning who had been waiting for a sober moment to witness to him and she made contact with him while I was on my way. I must tell you

I walked into that apartment in total expectation of not finding him alive. I really sensed this was the end. I was relieved to find him breathing, though the stench in the apartment was overwhelming. As a nurse and a Christian, I almost always sense death approaching.

He was sober, swollen and had much difficulty breathing, he refused my numerous urgings to call an ambulance stating he would refuse to go. I had had previous experience with those refusals so I knew that would be the case. I honored his wishes. I got him into the shower, it had to be with the assistance of angels I know. He's six foot weighing close to 300 lbs and I only 5'3". I changed the bed, dressed bed sores, and emptied emesis. I assisted him with drinking water because the tremors were so severe. He apologized to me, everyone, to God. I read him scripture, we talked about dying, we prayed and he repented and rededicated himself to Christ.

The day passed agonizingly slow and in the evening we watched a previous episode of "Touched by an Angel" unbelievably that night about unconditional love. The tremors and vomiting by this time worsened, his blood pressure was treacherously high, he still refused medical intervention. At one point in the episode, he crawled out of the chair over to me and shared loving thoughts that are private and to this day my heart cringes as I remember. He then leaned back against the chair. About one in the early morning hours exhausted I said to him I am so tired if you need me just call me. He misunderstood and asked me not to leave and I told him I had no intention of leaving I was just closing my eyes.

I awoke about two o'clock to a sound of gasping and a thud and ran to the bathroom. I checked for a radial pulse then carotid there was neither. I called 911 and then my friend. The paramedics confirmed what I already knew. His life here on Earth was complete. He was no longer suffering. The battle with addiction over!

We don't know the real depth of love until we are separated from it. A love that has been rekindled burns brighter when stirred. Our reconciliation was a rekindled love. Loving unconditionally will cost you. When storms stir the seas, and the forces of hell rise up intermittently in waves roaring toward the shore hitting with a violence enough to move the very foundation. When the blackness of night washes over you and you only see its destruction. You must search for the hidden treasure. His battle is over but the Victory won. I miss him terribly and though it has been almost two months the tears have not ceased as I write. They are fleshly tears of loss mingled with tears of joy that he is *with* the Lord. The darkest of the dark nights of my soul but the riches are not hidden.

The aftermath of the sudden death of a spouse is beyond description, sudden waves of despair appear without warning. They come roaring forth from nowhere when least expected. The very healing force is the most difficult ingredient of suffering. Time. Isaiah 61 tells of the coming of Christ to give me comfort, beauty for ashes and the oil of joy for mourning. One more treasure to look forward to. Better days will dawn just as I know the night will turn into day again. The pain will lessen, the tears will wash away the despair. I have been told weeping endures for a night but joy comes in the morning. I will not drown when the waves of emotion from deep seated loss come rushing at me with the force of a tidal wave threatening to engulf my spirit. I may go under for a brief moment but my lifeguard is there to rescue me pull me to safety. After all He said He would never leave nor forsake me.

When trembling rises up threatening to shake your very foundation and darkness threatens to engulf you, remember; the *Treasure* is hearing His voice in the winds of adversity ever so gently speaking to your heart. It is a ray of Son Shine like a silver shaft of light breaking through a storm darkened sky. The *Treasure* of life is found in Christ, The *Riches in Secret Places* unfolding the outcome of His divine plan hidden in the shadow of His hand. The *Secret*, is with them that fear {are in awe} and search for Him.

Epilogue in memory of: Michael Fred Lebendig, October 21,1950 to February 13,2010

Placed in my life by God that his love and challenging nature might help mold me into who I am today. A wounded heart like the rest of us, victimized by the circumstances of his past experiences but in the end finding victory and eternal life in Christ! You will forever be in my heart!

Acknowledgements:

My heartfelt gratitude and thanks to my patient, willing and loving grandparents: Hans and Josephine Sandvig who took me in as a small child initially shaping my spiritual walk. Pastors James and Janice Holder for the past fourteen years of spiritual parenting, my long-time friends and mentors Sister Sally Edgerly, Joyce Taylor and Rcv. Don Taylor who have provided love, support and challenging admonishment when needed. Clients, co-workers and friends who have offered the proving ground for experience and wisdom. Finally, my family and loved ones who without their patience, perseverance and love, I may never have completed this journey. God Bless You All!

And most especially to a loving faithful savior who from the beginning of time was always there to watch over me. Your faithfulness, mercy and grace is with me daily and my life is dedicated to serving you.

Author's Note:

If you have been touched by our stories and have not previously asked Christ into your heart, now is definitely an excellent time to experience a miracle change in your life, Take the opportunity now while you have the chance.

Prayer:

Heavenly Father, I come before you in the precious name of The Lord Jesus Christ. I believe that you suffered and died that I might have eternal life. I renounce all my past sins, known and unknown and profess from this day forward your Lordship over my life!

LaVergne, TN USA
30 July 2010
191574LV00003B/2/P

9 781609 573836